Patañjali's Yoga Sūtras

Gateway to Enlightenment
Chapter One

Rama Jyoti Vernon

LIGHTHOUSE
PUBLISHING

Portland, OR USA

Layout Designer: Mira Murphy

Editor: Ginny Beal

Illustrations: © 2017 Rama Jyoti Vernon

Publisher: Ann Wagoner

ISBN: 978-0-692-95887-2

Library of Congress Cataloging in-Publication Data

Cover photo: 123RF

For more information:

LIGHTHOUSE
PUBLISHING
925 NW Davis Street
Portland, OR 97209 USA
503-890-2105
www.lighhouseayurveda.com
ann@lighthouseayrveda.com
Printed in the United States

Table of Contents

Foreword i

Introduction..... I
- The Philosophical Systems of India IV
- The Three Guṇas VIII
- Six Paths of Yoga XII
- Patañjali and the Buddha XIII
- Overview of the Four Chapters of the Yoga Sūtras XV
- Beginning the Journey of the Yoga Sūtras XXIII

Chapter One: SAMĀDHI PĀDA
- Verse 1: Now we begin 1
- Verse 2: Understanding the mind 2
- Verse 3: The Seer and the Seen 20
- Verse 4-11: Waves of the mind 22
- Verse 12-16: Five non-painful waves of the mind 58
- Verse 17-21: Concentration & varying states of Samādhi 69
- Verse 22: Different practices and constitutions of students..... 77
- Verse 23-26: Īśvara 79
- Verse 27-29: Om and Īśvara 89
- Verse 30-33: Overcoming obstacles 94
- Verse 34: The importance of exhalation 100
- Verse 35-40: Other ways to still the mind 102
- Verse 41-51: Samādhi 108

Appendices
- Acknowledgments 131
- Recommended Reading 133
- Guide to Pronunciations 141

Foreword

I feel deeply honored to write this foreword. I've known Rama for over thirty years. She is widely respected and often referred to as the "Mother of Yoga in America." Her wisdom that comes from within ... a well that is always full!

Rama lives her life as a fountain of beneficence. Her generosity and creative energy spearheaded [or helped spearhead] a movement that brought yoga Masters and their teachings to the United States. *Yoga Journal Magazine* was a collaboration birthed at her own kitchen table.

Rama's lifetime of devotion to study with yoga practitioners in India and elsewhere is only one reason, her knowledge is so vast. She reminds us that enlightenment is not a destination, but a journey, wherein we may relax and "be here now." Rama writes with exquisite prose directing us to discern how heart-love is a treasure defined and shared in the *Yoga Sutras of Patañjali*, and how ever-expanding love leads to tranquility of mind. The present moment is a perfect place and time to begin, to be, and to breathe!

Having read Rama's book, I awakened to realize that we have in our hands a treasure, a book offering a deeper and more profound understanding of the psychology and practice of yoga than ever before.

Hopefully, we will learn in her next book — a long-awaited autobiography — about the years Rama spent resolving conflict between warring factions. She led 57 "Citizen Diplomacy" trips into the former Soviet Union, the new republic of Russia and many into the Middle East where she helped work on a conference between Arabs and Israelis.

My late husband Paul von Welanetz and I met Rama in 1985 when we traveled with her and a group of eighty into the Soviet Union. It was unprecedented! The first group of its kind. Our purpose was to film a documentary of "citizen diplomats" including peace activists Swami Satchidananda, actors Dennis Weaver and Mike Farrell, Dr. Patch Adams, author Alan Cohen, and futurist Barbara Marx Hubbard, to open an ongoing dialogue of peace between Russia and the United States. As I was packing the evening before our departure, a dear friend telephoned and asked why I was weeping. I answered from a deep knowing, "Our lives will never the same . . ." That trip indeed altered the trajectories of my marriage and the lives of so many others.

Throughout all the challenges of managing such a journey during the height of the Cold War, Rama was a vibration of serenity and inner peace. There are some who run from a conflict, some who run to fight, but so few who approach conflict offering a higher state of consciousness that actually opens dialogue and awakens true connection and compassion. Gorbachev said, "It was groups like hers, not just leaders, that helped end the Cold War."

Expecting a stern welcome, we were amazed to meet generous and heartfelt people. We rode the metros and taxis and lovingly connected with the locals when we got lost. Which was often. We met members of "Peace Committees" who had been completely closed to each other because of ethnic and political differences. Rama encouraged all to open their hearts and minds, and to share personal stories that led us all into deeper understanding and compassion. Paul and I returned home to completely reinvent our shared careers into one that became much more meaningful and beneficial to the world.

What is the secret to Rama's magical knowledge of conflict resolution? *Yoga!* Chapter One of her new book on the Yoga Sutras hands us the very threads that lead to tranquility of mind.

Reader beware: Many of those who have come to know this book, either in the capacity of editing, transcribing, copy editing, fact checking, organizing, publishing or designing have found their world changed to their great benefit.

Considering her history and contributions, one would wonder why Rama's name is not a household word. Being a naturally humble woman, Rama does not network, self-promote, nor market herself. She simply follows her inner guidance and trusts life to light her way. So, we are fortunate indeed to be discovering this new book, her masterpiece.

Looking back over my seventy-five years, I see clearly how Paul and I became the founders of an organization that hosted, and had as members, many of the most inspiring and pioneering authors in the world for over thirty-three years. YES! I recognize and give thanks for how influential this radiant woman has been in so many lives.

More than anyone I know, Rama lives the words she speaks. Her knowledge has been both acquired and arisen from within—and it is sure to transform the world for generations to come.

Diana von Welanetz Wentworth

Diana von Welanetz Wentworth is the author of seven best-selling and award-winning books and the coauthor of two *Chicken Soup for the Soul* titles. Film rights to her romantic memoir, *Send Me Someone*, were purchased by the Lifetime Network. With her late husband Paul von Welanetz, she hosted a long-running television series and founded the Inside Edge (www.InsideEdge.org), a weekly breakfast forum in Southern California that helped launch the careers of many of the most celebrated authors and speakers of our day including Jack Canfield, Dr. Susan Jeffers and Louise Hay. Progressive business leaders still gather at the Inside Edge to discuss new ideas in psychology, science, global issues, success strategies, spiritual awareness and the arts.

Introduction

I have found the *Yoga Sūtras* to be the heartbeat of *yoga*. By incorporating them into my teachings over the past 50 years, I have learned that we cannot separate our *yoga* practice from the scriptures of the *Yoga Sūtras.*

Patañjali's *Yoga Sūtras*, which are said to be over 5,000 years old, are a great treatise on *yoga* and one of the deepest forms of psychology in the world today. To explore the future of modern psychology we have only to reach into our ancient past in *yoga*. The *Yoga Sūtras* are a map for our lives as well as a bridge between eastern and western studies of the human psyche.

To explore the future of modern psychology we have only to reach into our ancient past in yoga.

The teachings of the *Yoga Sūtras* are important for *yoga* practitioners because the verses give the reason *why* we are practicing *yoga*. The essence of all *yoga* can be found in the second *sūtra*, "*Yogaś Citta Vṛtti Nirodhaḥ,*" which means *yoga* is to still or quiet the turbulence of the mind. There are four chapters with 195[1] brief succinct aphorisms that give a definitive and sequential roadmap for how this can be accomplished. This original premise supports the conclusion and vice versa. They are systematically logical and, for this reason are known as the "Science of *Yoga*." Each *sūtra* rolls into the next like a beautiful story unfolding before us, explaining, redefining and adjusting to various students' character and tendencies. They lead into the inner sanctum of the human mind and soul. The *Yoga Sūtras* are the deepest psychology that, after thousands of years, still applies to our lives today. They can be woven into our practices of postures (*āsana*), breathing (*prāṇāyāma*), concentration (*dhāraṇā*) and meditation (*dhyāna*).

The *Yoga Sūtras* were not written but compiled from existing teachings passed on orally from *guru* to disciple in the ancient oral tradition of India. The *Āyurvedic* physician and Sanskrit grammarian named Sage Patañjali compiled them in a written form in approximately 250 CE. Therefore, he is known as the 'Father of *Yoga*.' Śri Patañjali condensed the existing teachings of *yoga* into a written outline form that is logical in its progression toward 'enlightenment.' This outline, known as the *Yoga Sūtras*, identifies the reasons for the pain we experience in our lives and gives a way out of that pain so that we may taste the freedom or liberation from the illusion of separation.

The term *sūtra* is from the Sanskrit root *su*, to thread or sew together and *tra*, in order to transcend. The *sūtras* thread together the pearls of ancient wisdom creating a necklace, rosary or Hindu *mālā* where the first bead is also the last, where after

[1] In the oldest and most classical treatise by Swami Hariharānanda Āraṇya, there are 195 *sūtras*, however in other later texts there are 196 *sūtras*.

touching each bead, one comes back to where they started. Just like the *mālā*, the *sūtras* form a circle or cycle of thought which follows a logical and sequential order. Everything in *yoga* should be like a *sūtra*, knotted together through relationship in a circle. In the words of B.K.S. Iyengar, "*Sūtra* means a thread. As the pearls are held on a thread, all the limbs of your body should be held on that thread which is called intelligence."

Each *sūtra* is like a *mantra*. *Man* means to think and investigate and *tra* means in order to transcend. Originally, they were to be repeated until the mind transcends itself and the meaning of each *sūtra* reveals itself to the aspirant. It was originally void of commentary, but now, we can revel in the multitudes of commentaries that are so readily available at this time on the planet. There are as many interpretations of the *Yoga Sūtras* as there are people. It is important to remember that even Patañjali compiled the *sūtras* from the vast storehouse of the *Yoga Śāstras* (scriptures) that are said to have existed since the beginning of time. Some of the commentaries are taken from a variety of other ancient scriptures such as *Sāṁkhya* philosophy and the Upaniṣads.

The commentaries in this book are meant to help the reader to integrate these teachings into their everyday life and into their *yoga* practice. This commentary is unique because it does not separate the philosophy from the practice of *āsana* and life. Over the past 50 years, the teachings of the *Yoga Sūtras* have guided and enriched my life, *āsana* practice and work in the international sphere. I have applied these teachings to conflict resolution between individuals and nations. I offer this commentary from my unique experience as a householder, a mother and a citizen of the world. This is not merely an intellectual study, but intended to give a glimpse into how to live the *sūtras* and use them as a roadmap through the many challenges we face in daily life.

My Journey with the *Yoga Sūtras*

I started practicing *yoga* when I was 15 years old in 1955. It was what I had been searching for as a child, to find a way out of emotional and physical pain to oneday experience inner peace. At that time, *yoga* was not widely known and there were only a few books in English on the subject. Later, when I was married, it was Mr. B.K.S. Iyengar who sent me to his book dealer in Pune, India. He gave me what I consider to be the most in-depth and esoteric commentaries on the *Yoga Sūtras* by Swami Hariharānanda Āraṇya. It was the *Yoga Sūtras* that gave me a deeper and broader understanding of how and why we practice *yoga* and how they could be incorporated directly into the postures of our life. I found that I could not separate the *yoga* poses from the poses of daily life. All *āsanas* were *mudrās* that are the gesture of the mind expressing itself through the body. If I changed the quality of my poses, I noticed a definitive correlation to the postures in my life. In short I discovered that the way we do our pose is the way we do our life and that the reflection of one was in the other.

Using the *Yoga Sūtras* to guide my practice has gradually led me to living a more harmonious and grace-filled life with momentary glimpses into the many ways in which the Divine manifests. I have found the inner experiences that have unfolded over the years described in the *sūtras*. The *sūtras* seemed to confirm the validity of these experiences.

The *Yoga Sūtras* led me to develop an International Peace Curriculum that incorporates the *sūtras* within conflict resolution from its personal psychological roots, and how this relates to our interpersonal relationship with others. For years, I worked in other countries effecting dialogue and conflict resolution roundtables with warring factions of countries using the *Yoga Sūtras* as an infallible guide. The *sūtras* guided my practice, my life and my work in teaching *yoga* teachers. Then I applied them in workshops in Global Citizen Diplomacy in regions such as the former Soviet Union, Afghanistan, China, Cuba, South Africa, Ethiopia and the Middle East (Israel, West Bank and Gaza).

I am so thankful that I have had master teachers over the past 50 years who have given me a key to unlocking the code of the *Yoga Sūtras* to see how they are a living, breathing organism that is timeless and eternal. The *sūtras* live within each cell of my being as I practice them in *āsana*, in every breath, in how I lift out of spinal compression to hold the higher mind consciousness where it is possible to discern differences without comparing those differences. The *sūtras* have taught me over the years that it is the *ego* part of my mind that loves to compare, which creates continual separation, not integration and unification. The *Yoga Sūtras* have brought me to an understanding beyond the words and beyond the forms of this three-dimensional world. Here I can catch glimpses into the unseen worlds beyond the human eye. They have given me the courage to transcend fear, and at times to step off the precipice of consciousness leaping into the unknown with only the wings of faith.

The *sūtras* have given me the courage to explore ever-new depths of the inner Universe and through their practices, soar to new heights of understanding and compassion. They have helped increase my understanding of human nature and the human heart. They have brought me into new unfolding experiences of non-criticism and non-judgment to find the one light that shines in all.

The Yoga Sūtras have brought to me an understanding beyond the words and beyond the forms of this three-dimensional world. They have helped increase my understanding of human nature and the human heart to find the One Light that Shines in All.

The Six Philosophical Systems of India

Yoga is one of the six philosophical systems of India, and Patañjali's *Yoga Sūtras* are one of the earliest treatises among them. The scriptures of *yoga* are like the threads woven into the tapestry of all six systems of Indian philosophical thought. It would be difficult to separate their teachings from all the others.

These six treatises are known as the *Ṣad Darṣanas*. *Ṣad* means six and *darṣanas* is from the Sanskrit root verb *dar*, which stems from '*driṣ*' meaning to see not just the form, but also the Universal energy behind the form and '*na*' a noun describing the 'eternal cosmic vibration.' *Ṣad Darṣanas* would then mean there are six ways of seeing the Divine behind the words or forms of the scriptures.

In these *Ṣad Darṣanas*, there is conspicuous absence of any mention of historical dates in ancient Indian treatises. This makes their chronological placement extremely difficult. The dates given are estimated by several sources but no one knows for sure. These systems can be found in different orders according to various scholars. I am listing them in the order in which I have been taught throughout the years.

I. VAIŚESHIKA: The Atomic theory of Creation

The word *vaiśeṣa* means 'attributes' and 'forms' and this philosophy is the study of the physical, atomic matter. *Vaiśeṣika* is a non-theistic philosophy that views the world as matter that is comprised of subatomic and atomic particles that come together to create composites that are viewed as matter and solidity. In this philosophical system, knowledge and understanding are achieved by studying the world and its matter. The world can be understood through studying the smallest bits of the universe (atoms and nuclear physics) or the formation of the largest galaxies (astronomy and the big bang).

The exponent of this system was Kanāda, who formulated these tenants in 300-600 B.C. He described nine fundamental categories of substances (mind, soul, time, space/direction, earth, water, air, ether, light) and the earliest version of atomic theory. Substance was described as one six categories of existence. This system studied the energetic movements of electrons, protons and neutrons way before we had the modern scientific terms for these subatomic particles. In *Vaiśeṣika*, the subatomic particles relate to the three *guṇas*, or constituent principles of creation. *Guṇḍ* means to bind and the *guṇas* are the binding force of the subatomic particles. The concept of the three *guṇas* is woven throughout all the *Yoga Sūtras*. In India these three binding factors of creation relate to the Hindu trinity of Brahma, Viṣṇu, and Śiva, respectively the Creator, the Sustainer, and the one that dissolves existing structures for the new to come forth.

The three *guṇas* are:

1) *Rajas* – activity, which relates to Brahma and the positive charge of the proton
2) *Sattva* – equanimity, which relates to Viṣṇu and the neutral charge of the neutron
3) *Tamas* – inertia, which relates to Śiva and the negative charge of the electron

The dance of Śiva can be seen as the frenetic dance of the electrons trying to free themselves from the bind of attraction to the positive charge of the proton. This creates the dynamic tension that is the dance of life. This is also the dance of the trinity Godhead between creation, sustenance and dissolution, all within each atom of our universe.

Modern researchers in a scientific laboratory in Illinois where subatomic particles are accelerated and studied, discovered a particle that 'binds' together the electron, proton, and neutron. They call this particle a gluon. The ancient Sanskrit word *guṇa* means *to bind*.

The understanding of the physical world through contemporary physics has advanced beyond what the *Vaiśeṣikas* may have ever dreamed possible, through discoveries of quarks, muons, leptons, neutrinos, pions, photons, kaons, quantum field theory, string theory and minute particles such as the Higgs boson that may or may not have mass. Physics is changing with continual new discoveries from the Large Hadron Collider at the CERN laboratory in Switzerland, and other detectors that sense gravitational waves in which time speeds and slows, and black holes collide. Physicists of today are studying the world in the *Vaiśeṣikas* tradition and have taken it to new horizons.

Vaiśeṣikas can relate to the *sūtras* through the understanding of the three *guṇas* and how the interaction of the *guṇas* creates the oscillations that cause the mind waves, which are concepts found in the second *sūtra*.

II. NYĀYA: The school of Logic

Nya in Sanskrit comes from *ni* meaning to lead and *ya* is the suffix that emphasizes the preceding verb. So *Nyāya* means to *really* lead from one sequential thought to another.

This school was founded in approximately 550 B.C by Gautama (not to be confused with Gautama Buddha) and taught rules for logic, rhetoric and causation, and proposed a general theory of knowledge. *Nyāya* gave rise to the philosophy of language and linguistics. *Nyāya* is also non-theistic and based on the science of logic that every conclusion must support its original premise, and the original premise must support the conclusion. It is a circle (*mālā*) of thinking in the *Yoga Sūtras* where the ending supports the beginning. Logic throughout the ages is based upon *Nyāya*.

In *Nyāya*, the ways of inquiry to gain valid knowledge are through direct perception, indirect perception, inference, comparison and reliable testimony from experts. This would be found in *Yoga Sūtra*, I:7, where Patañjali outlines the non-painful mind waves, which include perception, indirect perception and inference.

The *Yoga Sūtras* follow this logical equation of *Nyāya* and are known as a science because they are written in a logical and sequential manner in which one *sūtra* folds into the next and each succeeding *sūtra* builds its foundation on the one before.

III. SĀṀKHYA: Journey of Consciousness into matter

Saṁ means to put together with and *khya* means to enumerate or to *count. Sāṁkhya* is known as the numerical system of creation. This school was founded by Sage Kapila and elaborated by Īśvara Kṛṣṇa in 350 A.D. *Sāṁkhya* concerns itself with the numbers and descriptions of the categories of creation and existence. Its focus is the plurality of being and its methods emphasize discrimination within a dualistic framework: spirit (*puruṣa*) and matter (*prakṛti*). It is a non-theistic and dualistic philosophy based on realization through correct understanding of the principals of phenomenal reality.

This philosophical system is the basis of *yoga*. *Sāṁkhya* is the involutionary process of spirit incarnating into matter. It is based upon the interplay between *puruṣa* (pure consciousness) and *prakṛti* (primordial nature). *Puruṣa* is unmanifested, formless, immutable and unchanging; it is the substratum of being. *Puruṣa* is the masculine, Śiva, or the *Ha* (sun) in *haṭha yoga*. *Prakṛti* is primordial nature, the cause of material creation, which sparks the descent of consciousness into matter. *Prakṛti* is the feminine, Śakti, or the *ṭha* (moon) in *haṭha yoga*.

Knowledge is the result of interaction between the mind and the object. Nature and spirit, *prakṛti* and *puruṣa*, Śakti and Śiva, are the basis for *tantric* philosophy. The world that we see is the offspring of the marriage between spirit and nature. Spirit means the pure consciousness of *puruṣa*. The essence of nature is the energy of *prakṛti*.

> *"The divine marriage between nature and consciousness is when consciousness comes in contact with nature, nature changes."*
>
> *BKS Iyengar*

Prakṛti is the divine spark for all of creation; she can be seen as the dancing girl who reveals her charms in her dance for *puruṣa*. *Puruṣa* is enchanted and enticed into the dance of creation with her. The eternal dance of creation between Śiva, the *puruṣa* and Śakti, the *prakṛti*, plants the seed in the universal womb of creation and is birthed as the cosmic mind. *Prakṛti* is the Kuṇḍalinī Śakti, the dormant energy at the base of the spine that when awakened, opens higher centers of consciousness, that manifests in the human body as the libido. The libido is also the same energy that can be transformed into *kuṇḍalinī*. This vital creative force of energy is *prakṛti*.

When these two universal energies of masculine and feminine, *puruṣa and prakṛti,* come together, they create the sound of OM, the sound of creation. In Sāṁkhya philosophy sound relates to the ether element, which is space. Therefore, sound creates the space for all of matter to manifest. Out of this comes *mahat,* the cosmic mind or universal intelligence. *Buddhi*, individual intelligence or higher mind, grows out of *mahat* and from *buddhi* comes *ahaṁkāra*, the ego, or individual separative consciousness. Out of the union of *puruṣa* and *prakṛti* also comes the three *guṇas* (*sattva*-equilibrium, *rajas*-activity and *tamas*-inertia). The *sattva guṇa* gives rise to mind (*manas*) as well as the five organs of cognition (hearing, touch, sight, taste, smell) and the five motor organs (hands, feet, vocal cords, excretory and reproductive organs). The *tamas guṇa* gives rise to the *tanmātras* or the subtle states of the elements (sound, touch, vision, taste and smell) as well as the five elements themselves (ether/space, air, fire, water, earth) and these five elements give rise to all of matter. (See chart below.)

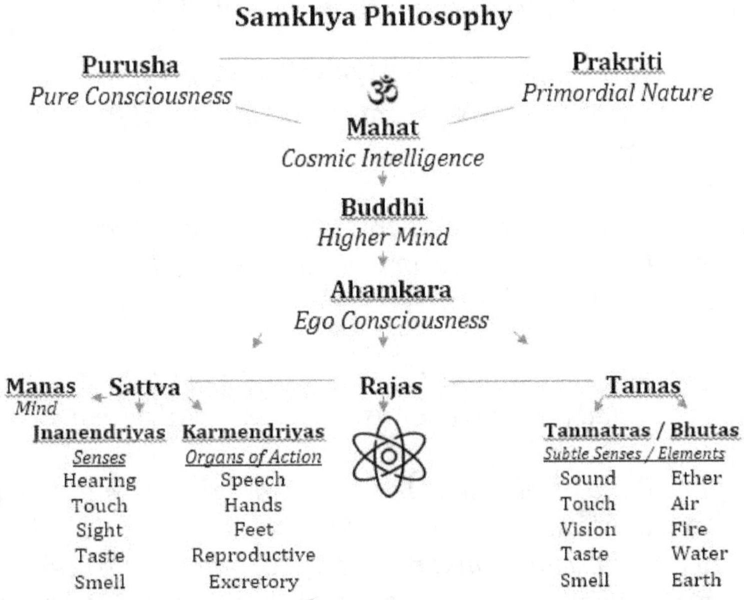

Sāṁkhya is the story of the involutionary journey of consciousness into matter. It is like an inverted tree with its roots in the heavenly spheres and its aspiring branches reaching into the density of earth elements. *Sāṁkhya* relates to the human form, and how the sensory organs and organs of locomotion give life to the physical body. *Sāṁkhya* has an involutionary as well as evolutionary perspective. It is the basis for *Āyurveda*. *Āyur* means life and *veda* means knowledge. *Āyurveda* is the knowledge of life, the Indian system of medicine and is based on *Sāṁkhya*. *Sāṁkhya*, *Āyurveda* and *yoga* are fundamentally linked.

The Three Guṇas

The three guṇas are concepts that interweave in and out of all 195 sutras in Patañjali's Yoga Sutras. They are foundational in the study of Yoga, Āyurveda or any Vedic study, so it is important that we take some time to describe them in more detail.

Guṇḍ means to bind. In Sāṁkhya philosophy, the guṇas are the constituent principles of creation that arise out of the union of puruṣa and prakṛti, out of Pure Consciousness and Nature. In Sāṁkhya philosophy, puruṣa, consciousness, exists in perfect harmony and equilibrium prior to joining with prakṛti. In the union with prakṛti, the spark of creation creates a friction that creates duality, out of this disequilibrium arise the three guṇas. They are energies that govern everything, from the subatomic particles to the galaxies in the Universe. They govern all life, through their magnetic and anti-magnetic fields that allow the electrons to encircle the protons and neutrons as well as the earth to rotate on its axis. They are the constituents that bind particles with gravity. These three guṇas are sattva, rajas and tamas (serenity, activity and inertia.)

***Sattva** is the principle of equilibrium, contentment, peace, harmony, and purity. It is the original state of the mind. This state of mind is ideal for spiritual practice.*

***Rajas** is the principle of movement and energy. It is associated with activity, restlessness, agitation, desire, aggression, will and self-seeking action. It has an outward motion.*

***Tamas** is the principle of inertia. It is associated with matter, density, dullness, obstruction, heaviness and darkness. It has an inward and downward motion.*

We can see the play of the three guṇas in any normal day. At night, when we sleep we are governed by tamas guṇa which causes the heaviness, darkness and the obstruction of our conscious mind necessary for the sleep state. In the morning when we arise and move out into the world to begin our activities of the day, we are governed by rajas, which causes motion and activity. Sattva is the basic state of the mind when rajas and tamas do not affect the mind. Sattva can be seen in our life in those quiet moments when the prāṇa, life force, is balanced between inward and outward motion, it is the equilibrium between all polarities. Many people experience a sāttvic state of mind through yoga and other spiritual disciplines. Many of the techniques of yoga are meant to bring us into a sāttvic state of mind.

IV. YOGA: Union

The *Yoga Sūtras*, a correlate of *Sāṁkhya*, were compiled by a physician and grammarian, the great Sage Patañjali who lived in the third century A.D. The Hindu tradition contends that Sage Patañjali was the incarnation of Ananta, Viṣṇu's thousand-headed Lord of the Serpents, the race that guarded the secret treasures of Earth. Some also believe that Patañjali is the same as the great *Āyurvedic* physician Caraka, the first scribe of the great *Āyurvedic* treatise, the *Caraka Saṁhitā*.

Yoga is derived from the Sanskrit verb '*Yuj*' meaning to yoke, harness, bind, fuse, join or bring together. *Yoga* as yoke can also be found in Middle English (yok), Old English (geo), Old High German (jok), Old Norwegian Gothic (yuk), Latin (jugum) and Greek (Zygon).

Yoga is commonly known as union—union of the individual with the universal; the Ātman with Brahman. It is union we are told, through the image of the oxen joined to its plow. It's a dynamic, not a static union. It can also be defined as reunion, communion, integration and reintegration of self with the universe, man with creation, material with the spiritual, the finite with the infinite, the individual with universal consciousness.

However, the great universal question is: Is it possible to join together that which has never been separated? Perhaps *yoga* is not 'doing' but 'undoing.' When Swami Satchidānanda was asked if he was a Hindu, he was silent and pensive for a moment and then said, "I think of myself as more of an 'undo.'" *Yoga* can be defined as a state of oneness or union as well as a methodology to bring the practitioner into that state. Its practice releases the impediments or veils that keep us from realizing that we are already one with the Universal Source.

When Swami Satchidānanda was asked if he was a Hindu, he was silent and pensive for a moment and then said, "I think of myself as more of an 'undo.'"

Yoga contains all the systems of Indian philosophical thought. The *Yoga Sūtras* are based upon the teachings of *Sāṁkhya* philosophy, which believes in self-realization through correct understanding of the principals of phenomenal reality and renunciation as well as integration of a worldly life. *Yoga* philosophy believes that no self-realization or knowledge of one's real self is possible without constant and disciplined practice of both mind and body. *Yoga* attempts to achieve this goal through the practice of societal and personal self-discipline, study of scriptures, meditation, *mantra*, *āsana* and *prāṇāyāma*.

The philosophical thoughts on spiritual liberation can be viewed as one whole thought system. It is obvious that *Sāṁkhya* and *yoga* are mutually complementary; one gives the theories and the other gives the instructions for the practice and how the theories can be experienced. The main treatise for this philosophical system is Patañjali's *Yoga Sūtras*. The *sūtras* contain all six philosophical systems within its verses.

Yoga is considered both theistic and non-theistic, whether *yoga* unites us with a divine higher power or whether it unites the microcosm of the individual with the macrocosm of the universal. *Yoga* is not a religion but is the essence of all religions. It is non-dogmatic, adapting its methods to fit the individual needs rather than expecting the individual to adapt to one way or belief system. *Yoga* is union, whether uniting with oneself, those around us, or a higher power.

V. PŪRVA MĪMĀṀSĀ: Ritual

Pūrva means whole, entire and earlier. *Mīmāṃsā* is from the Sanskrit root verb *man* to think or to investigate; it means inquiry into the revered scriptures of the Vedas.

Pūrva Mīmāṃsā was founded by Jaimini in approximately 200 B.C. It is a philosophy of ethical behavior and moral action that includes ritualism and priestly duties. *Pūrva Mīmāṃsā* is the early interpretations of Vedic texts that relate to *bhakti yoga*, the *yoga* of devotion, where intellect is transformed into higher intuition and emotions into devotion.

Mīmāṃsā held that the soul is omnipresent and focused on *dharma*. *Dharma* as it pertains to *Mīmāṃsā* school of philosophy means social and ritual duty. Although *Pūrva Mīmāṃsā* is non-theistic in its approach, it is theistic in its tenants of *bhakti*. It represents a non-Hindu approach to the *Upaniṣads*. The *Pūrva Mīmāṃsā* school emphasized *karma kanda*, the study of ritual action, whereas the *Uttara Mīmāṃsā* school of *Vedānta* emphasized *jñāna* (knowledge and wisdom) for understanding.

VI. UTTARA MĪMĀṂSĀ/VEDĀNTA: The Ending of Knowledge

Veda, meaning knowledge, comes from *vid* to pierce through or see and *anta* means the end, and can also relate to infinity where the end is also the beginning. So *Vedānta* is often translated as the 'ultimate end of knowledge,' but the deeper meaning refers to the beginning of what lies beyond knowledge. *Ut* means upward and *tar* from *tra,* in order to transcend. In *Uttara Mīmāṃsā*, we are transcending thinking and going beyond even mind.

Vedānta/Uttara Mīmāṃsā was formulated by Shankaracharya in 788 to 820 AD. Vedānta is based on the *Upaniṣads*, *Bhagavad Gītā* and the *Brahma Sūtras*, and some say Vedānta has been there as long as the *Upaniṣads*. They come together and coexist, because *Vedānta* incorporates the *Upaniṣads* from all four *Vedas* (*Ṛg*, *Yajur*,

Sāma and *Atharva*). Some believe Śaṅkarāchārya was a Divine reincarnation of Lord Śiva and he taught reality as a single indivisible whole.

Uttara Mīmāṃsā, or *Vedānta*, rises above dualistic thinking. It is fundamentally monotheistic, based on transcending the illusion of separation in the continual remembrance of the One Source. This philosophy contains within it, the nature of ultimate reality; Brahman is the Creator, Māyā is the illusion of separation, and Ātman is the individual soul. Theological schools of this system with their respective proponents are:

1) *Advaita* or the non-dualistic school according to Śaṅkarāchārya,
2) *Viśiṣṭādvaita* or qualified non-dualism according to Rāmānuja, and
3) *Dvaita* or dualist according to Mādhva

While *Pūrva Mīmāṃsā* focuses on ritual actions as a means to connect us back to the original source, *Vedānta* goes beyond action and even knowledge to continually hold the oneness out of which all creation flows. Lifting consciousness above the illusion of separation is *Vedānta*.

Vedānta and *yoga* weave in and out of each other as they both hold to oneness with creation. *Yoga* means to yoke or join with source. *Yoga* is *Vedānta* in that it brings the realization that we are not separate from the source, we are already one.

Note: Some consider the 7th philosophical system of India to be Buddhism while others consider it to be Integral Yoga as expounded by Śri Aurobindo Gosh.

INTEGRAL YOGA

Dr. Haridas Chaudhuri, a close disciple of Śri Aurobindo, felt that it was a possibility that *Integral Yoga* could one day be seen as the 7th philosophical system. *Integral Yoga*, or *pūrṇa yoga* as expounded by its founder Śri Aurobindo Gosh, represents the integration and affirmation of worldly life rather than withdrawing and negating society and the bustle of life around us. Stay in life and integrate spiritual practices into life. *Pūrṇa yoga* encourages one to face into and move toward life, remembering that we are in the world but not of the world.

Dr. Chaudhuri was a great philosopher and spiritual teacher who, like Swami Vivekānanda came from Bengal. Unlike Vivekānanda, he did not have the title Swami or wear the colorful ochre robes with a yellow sash, or the white flowing robes of Paramahaṁsa Yogānanda. However, this Doctor of Philosophy in his blue serge suits, was just as great a thinker on the Hindu texts who took the ancient teachings into a new age *yogic* revolution of his *guru*, Śri Aurobindo, who called it "*Integral Yoga*."

Dr. Chaudhuri could simplify volumes written by Śri Aurobindo, who I called the prophet of the new millennium. Just as in the time of Descartes who said, "I think, therefore I am," it was difficult for the minds of the time to grasp his brilliant and simple deductions. Śri Aurobindo was one of those spiritual giants whose visions stretched far beyond the past and the present into the future of humankind. He saw the spiritual potentiality of humankind and expanded the mind of his reader. I was one of those readers.

Dr. Chaudhuri would give me two or three pages to read on Aurobindo's *Integral Yoga* saying that we would discuss it in next week's lesson. I read it and mulled it over while cooking, cleaning, taking the children to school and still could not understand the words much less the concepts of Śri Aurobindo's integration of the various *Mārgas* or paths of *yoga*. It took me years to fully comprehend his unique approach that brought them together in a complete and all-encompassing synthesis and integration of one's consciousness into Divine Union.

Originally, I thought Śri Aurobindo's *Integral Yoga* was a radical departure from *yoga* as the path to seek one's own enlightenment, thus absconding from the illusion of this world. In his *Integral Yoga*, I began to realize that the state of 'enlightenment' was not an end in itself, but only the beginning. It was the beginning of a supra mental race of beings who would not leave this illusory world but transform it into a replica of the world where we were trying to get.

THE MĀRGAS: The Six Major Paths of Yoga

The term *Integral Yoga*, as founded by Swami Satchidānanda and espoused by many *gurus*, was usually the integration of the six major paths of *yoga* such as *rāja, haṭha, jñāna, bhakti, karma* and *tantra yoga*, uniting every aspect of the aspirant with God or the Absolute through every aspect of the personality: Action, Emotion, Will and Reason. Originally these paths were not separated, which can be found in the *Yoga Sūtras*. Patañjali never divided the mental of *rāja* from the physical of *haṭha yoga*. He never separated the intellectual of *jñāna*, from the devotional practices of *bhakti*. Nor did he separate the sound of *mantra* from the form of *yantra* which when combined is *tantra*, or *kuṇḍalinī yoga*. And of course, Patañjali did not separate these aspects of the human personality from the actions of life (*karma yoga*).

"Why did the paths of *yoga* become separated," I asked Dr. Chaudhuri. He answered, "Perhaps, the ancient sages believed that it was too much for one person to focus on all these paths and parts of the human personality at one time. If our psyche leans toward one tendency more than others, it is recommended that we start with that path that leads to the integration of the others. *Yoga* is really the integration of the human psyche." *Integral Yoga* implies an understanding of *yoga* in its completeness —an all-encompassing, all-aspected union with the Universal Self as God. We cannot leave a part of ourselves out of this union, through *yoga*. We must be able to unite with the Absolute through every aspect of our personality in a balanced and integrated manner.

> *We must be able to unite with the Absolute*
> *through every aspect of our personality*
> *in a balanced and integrated manner.*
> *Dr. Haridas Chaudhuri*

Patañjali and the Buddha

Those of us who have studied the *sūtras* as well as various forms of Buddhism, cannot help but see the comparison and parallel lines of thought between Buddha's teachings and the early commentaries on the *sūtras*. Because the *sūtras* contain no reference to the teachings or views of any other philosophical system, and because the *sūtras* do no refute the views of other systems as later philosophical writings do, it is assumed that the *Yoga Sūtras* preceded the advent of Buddhism.

It is believed that the commentaries on the *sūtras* were compiled around 250 CE after the spread of Buddhism in around 500 BCE. Perhaps this is why there are so many similarities in the commentaries of the *sūtras* and the teaching of the Buddha. This was at the time the Buddha was still seeking wisdom from the wise teachers as to the nature of life. Where have we come from? Why we are here? Where we are going? What are the secrets of birth, old age and death? As the Buddha searched in his pilgrimage for the nature of reality, it brought him to the feet of his teacher, Arada Kalima, a known *Sāṁkhya* philosopher of his time.

The *Yoga Sūtras* were passed from guru to disciple or teacher to student. The oral tradition was prevalent in the ancient days in an age when very few were able to read and write. For this reason, it was important that the *sūtras* be brief.

With the passage of time, the scriptures became scarce as the transmission of teachings required dedicated commitment, disciplined study and strict habits of life. These teachings would have become extinct if it were not for subsequent thinkers and scribes who kept the scriptures alive through their written commentaries.

Patañjali was one such scholar. He was a sage and grammarian who compiled existing teachings of *yoga* into brief aphorisms we now know as the *Yoga Sūtras*. These aphorisms frame the *Sāṁkhya Yoga* philosophy.

Caraka, author of the great treatise of *Āyurvedic* medicine, the *Caraka Saṁhitā*, is not just the name of the physician himself, but means wanderer. Whether that title referred to a great wandering physician, or the wandering organizational nature of the text, we do not know. While the true identity of Caraka is in question, some hold firm that the *Āyurvedic* physician Caraka and the sage Patañjali are one and the same.

At the time of the spread of Buddhism, it was an age of sharing knowledge including philosophy and medicine. Many Buddhist pilgrims spread knowledge across the lands, and *Āyurveda* extended across the East creating the foundation of medicine systems in Tibet, China, Thailand, Mongolia and even Greece out of which our western medical system was born. Whether or not Patañjali is the great wandering physician Caraka, we know there is a deep relationship between *Yoga*, *Āyurveda*, Buddhism and *Sāṁkhya*.

From the above six philosophical systems we can see how *yoga* is interwoven with all of them. This can be seen throughout the four chapters of the *Yoga Sūtras*. Before moving forward into expounding upon *yoga* we must understand the roots of knowledge, cultivated by great sages of the epochs and all the systems of thought and practice that have guided individuals for thousands of years.

> *"Sūtra weaves within a posture like a thread – like a string of pearls. The sūtra thread minds us, woven to a central theme; awareness of Self. Every part of the body is like a pearl, every part wedded to the Self."*
>
> *-BKS Iyengar*

OVERVIEW OF THE FOUR CHAPTERS OF THE YOGA SŪTRAS

I. SAMĀDHI PĀDA: On Concentration

Saṁ means to sum it up or put together with.
Adhi means to adhere to, stick to it unwaveringly (referring to mind).
Pāda is piece or little part. In this instance it means chapter.

Samādhi is becoming one with all. It is the ultimate concentration where subject fuses with the object. This *pāda* (piece) of the *Yoga Sūtras* illumines the view of the mind and how to become unwavering in the oscillations of the mind waves. This section is for the *sāttvic* practitioner who does not study with the intellect but has insights through intuition.

The *Yoga Sūtras* are all based on a system of understanding the mind (*citta*) and how the practitioner can bring the mind to one-pointed quietness through continual practice and non-attachment (*jñāna yoga*). The essence of all *yoga* can be found in the second *sūtra*, *"Yogaś Citta Vṛtti Nirodhaḥ"* meaning that *yoga* is to still or quiet the turbulence of the mind. Any reference to the body through practices such as *prāṇāyāma* and *āsana* (*haṭha yoga*) are given as a way to understand and quiet the mind (*citta*) and the impulses (*vṛttis*) that arise within its field.

Samādhi Pāda offers an understanding of the four parts of mind and how they relate to the way we view and process the experiences we call life. The four parts of mind (*citta*) are:

1) *Manas* – conscious mind,
2) *Citta* – subconscious mind (includes the entire field of the mind),
3) *Buddhi* – higher illumined mind, and
4) *Ahaṁkāra* – ego mind or separative consciousness.

The ancient commentaries of the *Yoga Sūtras* say that every subconscious impression was once a conscious experience and that every conscious experience becomes a subconscious impression. The interaction of these four parts of mind will determine the molecules of emotions that are an outgrowth of the thought waves or *vṛttis* that contribute to either turbulence or serenity. The meaning of *vṛtti* in Sanskrit literally means to come into existence and to rise upward.

Yoga practices in general, help to accelerate and bring up the impressions from the psyche (*saṁskāras* and *vāsanās*) from the deepest layers of the subconscious mind (*citta*) to the surface of the mind (*manas*) in a shorter time span than they would normally appear. *Yoga* delves into the psyche of stored emotions, bringing them to the surface of the conscious mind where they can be seen and in turn, released. Esteemed teacher, Mr. B.K.S. Iyengar taught us that the invisible must become visible before it can be eradicated or transformed. This process is the inspiration behind Śri Aurobindo's definition, "*Yoga* is compressed evolution."

Depending upon which part of the *citta*, or field of mind is operative will depend upon the way in which the non-painful or painful *vṛttis* manifest and express themselves. The *sūtras* do not mention emotions, but instead go to the origin and source of emotions, which are the mind waves or *vṛttis*.

Samādhi Pāda of the *Yoga Sūtras* outlines the five non-painful *vṛttis*:

1) *Pramāṇa* – correct perception of the world, which is gathered through:
    a. direct experience
    b. indirect experience
    c. inference
2) *Viparyaya* – incorrect perception
3) *Vikalpa* – imagination
4) *Nidrā* – sleep (as in psychological sleep or physical sleep as an escape from reality)
5) *Smṛti* – memory

The *vṛttis* that arise within the field of the mind as waves in the ocean manifest in a number of ways, some of which are:

1) turbulent waves like a stormy sea,
2) calm surface with turbulent undertow, and
3) calm, placid, completely still waters with no undertow.

In the last state, even the tiniest pebble cast into its center cannot create a ripple of disturbance. This is what Patañjali refers to in the second *sūtra* as "*Yogaś Citta Vṛtti Nirodhaḥ.*" When the waves of the mind become still and calm, life's 'pebbles' or 'boulders' will be felt, but will not create waves, nor a pretense of calm on the surface with suppressed undertows beneath. Dr. Haridas Chaudhuri, founder of the California Institute for Integral Studies used to say, "Be like the rock off the shores of the ocean, feel the waves playing upon you, but stay centered in *yoga* so the waves will not knock you over. Be like the rock!"

In the state of "*Yogaś Citta Vṛtti Nirodhaḥ,*" one can look from the placid surface to the depths of mind that are free from any undertow and see the reflection of one's self. This is the state that Patañjali refers to in *Sūtra* I:3 as "*Tadā Draṣṭuḥ Svarūpe Avasthānam*" where "the seer and the seen become one."

After establishing the *yogic* view on the science of mind, Patañjali then gives a clear outline of the myriad of ways in which we can quiet the waves of the mind. He speaks of the three types of students, mild, medium and intense and how in each of these divisions there are also three methods: slow, medium and speedy. He gives several choices and methods for all types of students.

The first method he discusses is through continual practice, or checking the downward pull of body, mind and spirit, and detachment. Another approach lies within 'devotion to the lord of this world,' or *Īśvara*. With devotion and repetition of the name *Īśvara*, an aspirant can quiet and still the turbulence of the mind. Repeating "OM" and contemplating its meaning will help one realize the individual self and the obstacles will drop away.

Patañjali outlines the obstacles or impediments that disturb the mind (sickness, incompetence, doubt, delusion, sloth, instability to stay in a *yogic* state). These obstacles are daily occurrences in one's everyday life that keep us bound to this world of polarities and take continual vigilance to transcend.

He speaks in this chapter about sorrow, dejection and restlessness of body and how the instability of breath arises from a distracted mind. In this chapter, he emphasizes that the *yoga* practitioner can calm the mind by exhaling but he does not mention the practice of inhalation as a means to quiet the waves of the mind. If these still do not fit the aspirant, he gives several more suggestions finally saying we can calm the mind by whichever of these methods we may choose.

This chapter is a little more advanced than Chapter II because Patañjali discusses in detail the different stages of *samādhi*, which is the sustained *yogic* state of union. These states are outlined in a definitive way. This is the reason for the title of the Chapter, *Samādhi Pāda*. This is why some teachers recommend that some students of the *Yoga Sūtras* first read the second chapter on practice, *Sādhana Pāda*.

II. SĀDHANA PĀDA: On Practice

Sādhan means to go directly to the goal
na is the eternal cosmic vibration

Sādhana Pāda is the section that outlines the practices that take the aspirant to the goal of joining with the eternal cosmic vibration.

This is the chapter, some say, for the more *rājasic* or restless practitioner of *yoga*. If one cannot overcome the obstacles in the first chapter and quiet the waves of the mind, there are other suggested methodologies given. They continue to adapt to the nature of the aspirant. This first part of the chapter delves into the source of our pain and suffering in life. The second part gives us the practice of *yoga* to bring us out of our suffering. It defines *kriyā yoga* as discipline, study and surrender to a power beyond the limited self. It gives a compilation of moral, ethical and societal codes of behavior and then describes varying perspectives on the obstacles to *samādhi*.

In the first half of *Sādhana Pāda*, Patañjali encapsulates the origins of our pains in life that contribute to the turbulence of the mind, which keep us in delusion and separation. The sources of our pain lie within the five painful *vṛttis* called *kleśas*. *Kliś* means to inflict and *kleśas* are defined as afflictions. The five *kleśas* are:

1) *Avidyā* – ignorance, or not seeing the nature of our oneness,
2) *Asmitā* – egoism or identifying with limited individual consciousness,
3) *Rāga* – attachment,
4) *Dveśa* – aversion, and
5) *Abhiniveśa* – clinging to life and fear of death, or of the unknown.

Pain, be it physical or psychological, is an instrument that brings us to find a solution to the pain. We come to *yoga* when we *recognize* we are in pain. The practice of *yoga* brings up what is in the depth of the mind. It does not create the pain but merely reveals what is already there. Once uncovered it can be seen. It is in seeing alone that *kleśas*, the reason for our pain and suffering, are overcome and transcended. The word 'transcended' is used to simply mean to get on top of our pain. When we feel the sea of human suffering, it is possible to view ours in perspective. When that state is held, even the *vṛttis*, born out of *kleśas*, will arise and they will not have a hold on the practitioner. This is the state of mind known as *ekāgratā* (one-pointedness).

The seeds of the *kleśas* manifest in five evolutionary ways, from the dormant or repressed to the fully blown, then alternating state, to the thinned and finally scorched, where the aspirant is free from the downward pull of the mind.

In *Sādhana Pāda* we visit the subject of *karma*, or actions. *Karma* comes from the verb root *kri*, which means to do or to act and *ma* that is a primordial force of nature. *Karma* means actions and as we know, every action causes a reaction. It is the cause and effect cycle, giving birth to fruits that bear the same qualities as our past actions. There are three types of *karma*:

1) *Prārabdha* – The circumstances we are born into,
2) *Kriyamāṇa* – The karmas we are creating now. There are two parts:
    a. result of past actions that we are now experiencing and
    b. current actions that will determine future experience, and
3) *Sañcita* – Fruit of the past actions and the seeds of future experiences.

The second chapter of the *sūtras* catalyzes a broader view of the positive and negative effects of *karma* and how they can influence every phase of life and, according to ancient *yogis*, the lives yet to come. The *sūtras*, like the *yoga* practices, stress the importance of the latent unseen depths of the psyche through the subconscious mind and its cyclic reinforcement of cause and effect.

There is a powerful *sūtra* in this chapter that begins with a commentary, "We cannot avoid the pains of the past because they have already occurred. We cannot avoid the pains of this moment because they are in the process of occurring." Then the *sūtra* so brilliantly says, "*Heyaṁ Duḥkham Anāgatam,*" the only pain that can be avoided is the pain yet to come. This *sūtra* elucidates the reason why we seek out the healing benefits of *yoga*, whether it's physical, mental or emotional.

In the compressed evolution of *yoga*, we do not wait for the result of our past actions (*karmas*) to manifest, but consciously bring it up to the surface of the mind where we can see it, feel it, heal it, and in turn, release it. This is what is meant by B.K.S. Iyengar when he says, "The invisible must become visible before it can be eradicated."

A *yogi* is one who is accelerating the process of his or her own evolution by bringing up the various layers of impressions out of the latent depths of the psyche. These impressions have been produced by past actions (*karmas*). The *yoga* scriptures say that every subconscious impression was once a conscious experience.

Major *yoga* practices such as *āsana*, *prāṇāyāma*, *dhyāna*, *mudrā*, etc., are all meant to speed up our *karmas* by bringing the latent *saṁskāras* (impressions) or *vāsanās* (subtle impressions) that are stored in the physical and subtle nerve sheaths up to the surface where they can be seen. If we consciously see them, then we will no longer be a victim of our own mind waves. We will act instead of react.

The deeper and more subtle impressions (*vāsanās*) will lead to future actions and experiences. The *vāsanās*, in turn, lead to future *vṛttis* that lead to future actions (*karmas*). This is the never-ending cycle known as, "The law of cause and effect" and known biblically as, "What we sow, we shall reap."'

The second half of the second chapter gives five out of the eight progressive and sequential steps to eradicate or transform *kleśas* known as *Aṣṭaṅga Yoga* or the eight limbs of *yoga*. In this chapter, Patañjali gives the most commonly known aspect of *yoga* sometimes known as *rāja yoga* or 'the royal path' of *yoga*:

1) *Yama* – restraints
    a. *Ahiṁsa* – non-violence
    b. *Satya* – truthfulness
    c. *Asteya* – non-coveting
    d. *Aparigraha* – non-grasping
    e. *Brahmacarya* – regulation of the senses

2) *Niyama* – observances
    a. *Śauca* – purity of body and mind
    b. *Santoṣa* - contentment

c. *Tapas* – the fire of self-discipline
d. *Svādhyāya* – study of self through meditation
e. *Īśvara praṇidhāna* – surrender to God or 'higher self'

3) *Āsana*– postures
4) *Prāṇāyāma*– breath control
5) *Pratyāhāra* – withdrawal of senses

These five limbs are more commonly known and practiced in the field of *Yoga* and are said to appeal to the *rājasic* student, giving more concrete methods of practice to still the mind.

Yamas and *Niyamas* are the foundational codes of conduct that help the mind come into balance through favorable behavior. They humble the ego, which is important before progressing in *āsana*, which can create more power within the aspirant. *Yamas* and *Niyamas* are meant to precede *āsana* and also to be practiced within *āsana* and every phase of life.

Āsana, as one of the eight limbs, is meant to overcome the *kleśas* that manifest in the body. *Āsana* teaches us to hold the pose until one day — the pose holds us! *Āsana* is the most outwardly visible way to curb the restless *vṛttis* that manifest through the body's pains. It is through the practice of *āsana* that the practitioner can find comfort in all of life's positions, physically and emotionally. The practice of *āsana* is not meant to hold the pose…but to hold the *mind* through the pose.

One can condense and compress one's evolution, by diving deeply into the *āsanas* with the breath to bring up the painful experiences and memories of the past for their healing and releasing. This is reflected in the names of the *āsanas* that include the prefix *ut* or *ūrdhva,* meaning upward or *ṛi* meaning to rise upward. *Vṛtti* also means to come into exist and an impulse rise upwards. Through the practices of *āsana* we allow the pains buried in the deepest layers of the psyche to rise upwards to the surface of the conscious mind to be seen, felt and transformed.

The next sequential step after *āsana* Patañjali gives is *prāṇāyāma.* This is practiced after one achieves steadiness and balances the polarity of opposites through *āsana*. After this, the *Sūtras* say, one is fit for *prāṇāyāma*. The commentaries emphasize that *prāṇāyāma* practice with a restless mind produces further restlessness. It has also been found that *āsana* practice without the breath produces a restless mind. The essence of all *prāṇāyāma* is *kevala kuṁbhaka*, which means isolated and absolutely pure, where the in and out breath fuse into one another. In this state we are not breathing, but breath is.

Pratyāhāra is the next step from *prāṇāyāma*. When the mind is still and the in and out breath are happening simultaneously, there is a fusion that happens where the senses are automatically drawn inwards. *Pratyāhāra* cannot be forced or practiced but it is the outgrowth of the practice of *āsana* and *prāṇāyāma.*

Chapter II of the *Yoga Sūtras* gives growing awareness of how every conscious experience becomes a subconscious impression (*saṁskāra*). It delves deeply into the impact of those cellular memories upon our present and future lives. The positive and negative effects of *karma* help us to understand the consequences of our thoughts, words and actions. This chapter illuminates the source of our pains in life (*kleśas*) and outlines the practices to bring them to the surface of the mind so they may be transformed. *Yoga* is the method of eradication of the *kleśas* and it is done through the eight-fold path. The last three of the eight limbs are expounded in Chapter III, *Vibhūti Pāda*.

III. VIBHŪTI PĀDA: Supernormal Powers

Vi means to negate
Bhū is of the earth and *bhūta* means elements

Vibhūti Pāda is the section that negates the laws of the elements, moving beyond to a state where supernormal powers are attained.

This chapter is also known as *Saṁyama Pāda*. *Saṁ* is to sum it up or put together with and *yama* to restrain. It consists of the last three steps of *Aṣṭaṅga Yoga*:

6) *Dhāraṇā* – concentration,
7) *Dhyāna* – meditation, and
8) *Samādhi* – fusion and oneness of consciousness.

When Patañjali speaks of *dhāraṇā* he describes the varying stages of mind from the infatuated and obsessed, to the scattered, to the stillness of mind in *samādhi*.

These five states of mind are:

1) *Mūḍa* – dullness or apathy to one's own spiritual unfolding,
2) *Kṣepta* – scattered and turbulent, disarrayed, worrisome and fearful,
3) *Vikṣepta* – alternating state – sometimes turbulent and sometimes one-pointed and calm,
4) *Ekāgratā* – one-pointed where the same thought (*vṛtti*) that rises in the field of mind is replaced by the same or similar thought, and
5) *Nirodaḥ* – nothing can disturb the calm, the attainment of the state where the seer and the seen become one (I.3).

When *dhāraṇā*, *dhyāna* and *samādhi* are practiced simultaneously, it is known as *saṁyama*. This chapter deals with the *yogic* form of concentration and meditation. The *sūtras* are detailed in their description of the powers that come through *saṁyama* upon various energy centers of the body or anything that is inspirational. It discusses the types of 'powers' that manifest through specific focal points of concentration such as, "by practicing *saṁyama* on the sun, the point of the body known as the solar entrance, the knowledge of the cosmic regions is acquired."

It took me years to read Chapters III and IV of the *sūtras* because I felt I needed to study and practice the preceding chapters before I could understand the more esoteric verses. Apparently, the chapters of the *sūtras* are meant for the three types of students that Patañjali refers to as mild, medium and intense. I felt I was one of the mild ones, so it took years for me to gather the courage to delve into the third chapter of the *sūtras*, which is the exploration of the labyrinth of the mind, and what happens to the soul upon death. It speaks of the many *lokas* or worlds that our consciousness can enter into depending upon our spiritual understandings in this life. The *sūtras* are extensive in their exploration of the journey of the human soul after death and the many dimensions and *lokas* (worlds) that exist on an invisible and internal plane of consciousness.

This is an exciting chapter that shows possibilities and the power of the *yoga* practices. It honors the experiences of those who have preserved this body of knowledge throughout millenniums. Practice of the previous chapters gives a strong base and preparation for such 'powers' to manifest where the aspirant does not become attached but allows these experiences to come and go remembering that if certain powers should arise, they are a byproduct and not a goal or end in itself. In the last *sūtra* of this chapter, Patañjali says, "When equality is established between *buddhi* and *puruṣa*, in their purity, liberation takes place."

IV. KAIVALYA PĀDA: On Self-in-Itself or Liberation

Kevala means isolated and absolutely pure.

"Absolute consciousness becomes established in its own self." These last words of the previous *sūtra* support the original tenant of "*Yogaś Citta Vṛtti Nirodhaḥ*:" *yoga* is to quiet or still the fluctuations of the waves of the mind. This last chapter goes deeply into that state of liberation. It covers three major aspects of *karma* (action) and the *karmāśayah*, *saṁskāras* (subconscious impressions) and *vāsanās* (deeper latent impressions) that result in future *vṛttis*, desires and actions. The law of cause and effect is a major focal point of this chapter, even though it is mentioned in the second chapter. Also, Patañjali once more explains the *guṇas*, this time in more detail. He establishes the importance of discriminating between *buddhi* and *puruṣa*. "When one who has realized the *puruṣa*, inquiries about the nature of his or herself ceases."

This chapter is a synopsis of the previous chapters and a more in depth and expansive overview of all the previous *sūtras* bringing a more advanced approach. This chapter is so rich in its detail of the effects of our thought and actions, helping to remind the aspirant that non-attachment, or inaction within action brings the mind to one-pointed quietness and produces no future rebirths. This concludes the last chapter of 'Self-in-Itself 'or liberation of the *Yoga Philosophy of Patañjali.*

Beginning the Journey of the Yoga Sūtras

When you read and chant the *sūtras*, try to ingest them as you would your own breath. In the beginning of your study it helps to read several versions consecutively to get an idea of the difference in translations and concepts. This keeps your mind open and unattached and gives a broader understanding of the many paths to the same source.

If the study of the *sūtras* overwhelms you, take just one *sūtra* and/or commentary that has meaning for you and explore it, not just within its pages but also within the pages of your Soul. Repeat it in English or the phonetics of Sanskrit to yourself. Close your eyes and contemplate the meaning and value to you.

Our understanding and love of the *Yoga Sūtras* will continue to change and deepen with time and attention. Some of you will naturally feel more committed than others to this vast but simple study. For some, the meaning and understanding is immediate and for others it takes more time.

The importance of your own *sūtra* study is to prepare yourself by opening and offering yourself with love and reverence to the ancient wisdom that already flows through you. The *sūtras* remind us that we are already one with the eternal source of creation, that we are responsible for our own creations, and that we are *all* the architects of our own destiny.

> *The importance of your own sūtra study is to prepare yourself by opening and offering yourself with love and reverence to the ancient wisdom that already flows through you.*

SUMMING UP

The *Yoga Sūtras* are a practice and a way of life. They do not disappear when we close our book. They are not an intellectual study outside of ourselves but a study of ourselves. They are the deepest psychology that addresses the symptoms as well as the roots and origins of life's conflicts and difficulties.

The study of the *Yoga Sūtras* helps us not only to work through the "causes of our own sufferings" in life but also to work through the multilevel web of practices, techniques, and philosophies of *yoga* without seeing them as ends in themselves. The *sūtras* are not a study separate and apart from our every breath movement and thought, they give the reasons for our breath, our thinking process, our actions and reactions in this field we call life.

The study of the *sūtras* is like entering a hidden vault of the mind and all its chambers. It takes time to enter into its labyrinth. You can deepen your understanding each time you read over its sacred essence or discuss verses with others, meditate quietly upon specific verses and meanings, or feel their vibrations through chanting or repeating the sounds.

We may think of *Yoga* philosophy as something to study outside of ourselves, but the *Yoga Sūtras*, even though said to be thousands of years old, are the deepest psychology of the human mind. They are current today and give us a mind map of how we can realize the Self and realize the oneness of which we are already a part. Its teachings are a key for how to live each day of our life with greater awareness and understanding of universal laws and the refinement of our own inner evolutionary unfoldment. If we know how to incorporate The *Yoga Sūtras* into our lives of today, we will discover that the realization of oneself is not just on the mountaintops but in the everyday marketplace of the human soul.

If we know how to incorporate The Yoga Sūtras into our lives of today, we will discover that the realization of oneself is not just on the mountaintops but in the everyday marketplace of the human soul.

Invocation to the Supreme Deity

My homage to that being who is devoid of all misapprehension, free from the ME-feeling, above desire and anger, and bereft of all fear

My homage to Him who is in perfect quiescence and peace, calm, beyond all attachments, above all cravings, who has perfect knowledge of the metempiric Self and is self-contained

My outer self (the body) is in Thee; You are present in my inner self. Oh Lord, You manifest yourself in my inner heart free from all perturbations and worries.

Oh, Om! Om! Om! (Īśvara), my all is in You and You are present in my inner Self; please direct me to be mindful of Thee; may I be led by my spirit; may I have peace of mind.

May I, have constant remembrance of Thee and of my purified Self, dwelling only in Thee.
Oh, Om! Om! Om!

I.1 ATHA YOGA ANUŚĀSANAM

***Atha** = Now*
***Yoga** = union*
***Anu** = to flow along with*
***Śāsa** = śastras or scriptures*
***Nam** = to revere*

And Now, We Will Follow Along With The Scriptures of *Yoga* And Revere Them.

This first word of the first *sūtra, Atha* means now. It is no ordinary 'now.' It is a powerful statement meaning and *Now! A*ll that we have done, all we have experienced in this life and beyond that has brought us to this privileged point in time to hear and study the scriptures. "Now" is the convergence of our life's path, thoughts and actions that has brought us to this form of study, at this point in life. The *Yoga Sūtras* are a form of self-discovery that is not outside of your self, but is the study of the Self that can be incorporated into our everyday life. The Sanskrit word for "Now" may be over 5,000 years old, but it is a magnificent word that sums up our life, our interests in deeper studies of *yoga*, and it is the culmination of our internal journey on the path to the pathless land.

Yoga means to unite or to join. It is the union of *Ātman* with the *Brahman*, the individual soul with the Creator. However, if we look at it in a more universal perspective, *yoga* is not joining or bringing together. Instead, the practices of *yoga* are meant to release the impediments that keep us from realizing that we are already one.

Anu is a beautiful word. It means to flow along with the grain, not to interrupt, not to reverse the flow of that which is natural, but to flow along with. In this instance, it means to flow along with the scriptures of *yoga*.

The word *śāsa,* is an interesting word. It refers to the *śāstras*, which are the scriptures of *yoga*. *Śāstra* also means weapon. If we think about this, we will see that a weapon is something that is sharp where the energies are brought to one point. In this instance, it would be the point of piercing through the veil of illusion or separation. We use the scriptures to pierce through the veil of illusion.

The end of this word is *nam,* which means to revere or to have reverence for. Therefore, we can interpret this first *sūtra* as, "And now we will follow along with the scriptures of *yoga* and revere them."

This is a reverential beginning as we enter into the profound mystical and practical journey of the *Yoga Sūtras.* This *sūtra* is a reminder that honors the great masters that have preserved these ancient teachings for all future generations and millenniums to come. We pay homage and honor to the source that flowed through them giving us a vast insight into the ever-deepening teachings of *yoga*. This first verse prepares our minds and our hearts to receive the blessings of the great Ones who have walked before us, clearing a path to a gateway of enlightenment.

I.2 YOGAŚ CITTA VṚTTI NIRODAḤ

Yoga *= from 'yuj' meaning to yoke, harness, join, bring together or unite*
Cit *= to collect*
Citta *= mind as well as the subconscious mind*
Vṛ *= to come into existence or rise upwards, impulses*
Vṛtti *= electrical impulses that arise in the field of the mind; to come into existence*
Ni *= negates*
Rodhaḥ (Rudra) *= God of storms, in the Vedas*
Nirodaḥ *= without storms in the mind*

***Yoga* Is To Still Or Quiet The Storms Or Impulses (Waves) That Arise In The Field Of The Mind.**

NOTE: Other translations say, "Yoga is the suppression of the modifications of the mind." I do not use this definition because I do not use the word suppression. This word implies repression, which is the opposite of the intent of our yoga practice.

This *sūtra is* the most important part of the *Yoga Sūtras*; it is the essence of all yoga. It is the reason why we practice. The *Yoga Sūtras* are all based on a system to understand the mind. This is why we are practicing yoga. Any reference to the body through practices such as *prāṇāyāma* and *āsana* are given as a way of understanding and quieting the mind (*citta*) and the impulses (*vṛttis*) that arise within its field.

Mental fluctuations manifest, as thoughts and the effect of unbridled thoughts are emotions. Agitated thought distresses the system and deprives it of light, creating compression and depression, which turn inwards and contract with negative thoughts. We pull in like a black hole, which absorbs light, emitting very little from it.

CITTA - The Mind

The word *citta* is derived from the verb *cit*, which means to collect and *citi,* which refers to super-consciousness. The reflection of *citi* on the individual soul is called *citta*. Therefore, *citta* is an instrument or medium through which the individual soul relates to the world and evolves until it has become perfected. *Citta* is considered to be a bridge between the individual soul and the Divine Reality (God).

The *vṛttis* are disturbances on the *citta*, which are the cause of confusion, illusion and delusion. In the ocean, the waves are created by the wind in the same way the *citta*, the mind waves, are created by the *vṛttis*. The *vṛttis* are created by our emotions of anger, hate, happiness, pleasure, pain, repulsion and attraction. The mind waves are innumerable. This *sūtra* reminds us to gain voluntary control over them, to quiet the waves by bringing them into stillness (*nirodaḥ*).

Citi equals the Self, which is without any *vṛtti* or thought waves. When thought waves appear it becomes *citta*. So to unite with *citi* we are stopping thought waves. If there is no ocean there are no waves. Patañjali does not say to dry out the ocean but to stop the waves.[1]

Citta is used to refer to the entire mind, which according to the *Yoga Sūtras* consists of four parts. *Citta* also implies one part of the mind known as the "unseen" or subconscious mind. The mind oscillates between four functions. The four parts of mind are:

1) *Manas*
Manas is the part of the mind that gathers the impressions brought in by the five senses of perception.

2) *Citta*
Citta is the storehouse of impressions from previous conscious experiences. It is considered to be unseen and thus relates to the subconscious mind. Every conscious experience becomes a subconscious impression.

3) *Ahaṁkāra*
Ahaṁkāra is the ego, which separates, categorizes and compares differences. It is unlike the *buddhi* that sees the differences without judging. The ego compares those differences — 'I like this, I don't like that.' When ego is involved in rationalization or intellectual evaluation, it presents judgments in favor of its own demands.

4) *Buddhi*
The *buddhi* is the over-mind, sometimes called the higher mind, which witnesses and sees objectively. It is discerning. It sees differences but does not compare those differences. It is like a filtering machine, letting only refined impressions move deeper into one's being

How do these four parts of mind interact?
If the *citta* or subconscious is filled with negative impressions it taints the ego, *ahaṁkāra,* making it unhealthy. This means abnormal attachments, cravings, infatuations, un-satiated desires, and possessiveness. An unbalanced subconscious makes the intellect almost subservient to the interests of *ahaṁkāra*, ego. Our intellect, instead of being assisted in the process of integration and understanding becomes a hindrance and leads to unclear function of the mind and the senses (*manas*).

On the other hand, if the storehouse of impressions in the *citta* are brought to the light of the conscious mind, and seen, felt and transmuted, wisdom arises. When wisdom, *buddhi*, dominates the four parts of mind, a*haṁkāra*, ego, is sublimated in service of higher will.

---

[1] *From Rama's notes from the silent sage, Baba Haridas*

And now we will explore these four parts of mind in more depth:

MANAS – Conscious Mind

Man means to think. *Manas* is the thinking mind. This is the conscious part of mind that receives sensory impressions. Our five primary senses – sight, smell, hearing, taste and touch are often called the gateways to perception. We receive information through our senses but like all effective gateways, they are narrow and don't allow everything to enter at once. The job of the sensory organs, eyes, ears, nose, tongue and skin is to organize and translate the massive quantity of information we receive from the outside world into manageable bits of data. Without this way to control the barrage of incoming data, we would be constantly overwhelmed and exhausted. It is speculated that the brain processes between 50,000 and 70,000 thoughts a day (35 to 48 thoughts per minute).

Our senses represent less than one tenth of what is actually going on around us, such as the earth spinning and rotating on its axis, the movement of subatomic particles in the universe or the myriad of biochemical processes within the body.

Manas influences the sensory perceptions and gathers the impressions, which determine how we perceive a situation; how we take in facts or "reality." This part of the mind receives the sense impressions and forwards them to the intellect for evaluation, assortment, organization and rejection. And while a portion of the impressions brought by the senses is studied, a remaining part passes into the *citta*.

CITTA - SUBCONSCIOUS MIND

Cit means to collect, and like its name, it is a storehouse of the impressions that are gathered and caused by the other parts of the mind. *Citta* is the subconscious that is responsible for recollection, memorization and mental retention. In the practice of *yoga* disciplines, it is the subconscious that plays the greatest role because a profound change in personality cannot be brought about until the subconscious is overhauled and its impressions brought to the surface of the mind where they can be experienced and in turn, eradicated or transformed. The essence of *yoga* is to make the invisible become visible. The Greek philosopher Plato observed in 440 B.C. that the invisible is greater than the visible. It is in the realm of the invisible that we as humans have the greatest impact on our own destiny and wellness.

> *"You must bring the unconscious into the conscious. Intensified action brings intensified intelligence"*
>
> *- B.K.S. Iyengar*

Pyramid of the Subconscious Mind (citta) to the Conscious Mind (m*anas*)

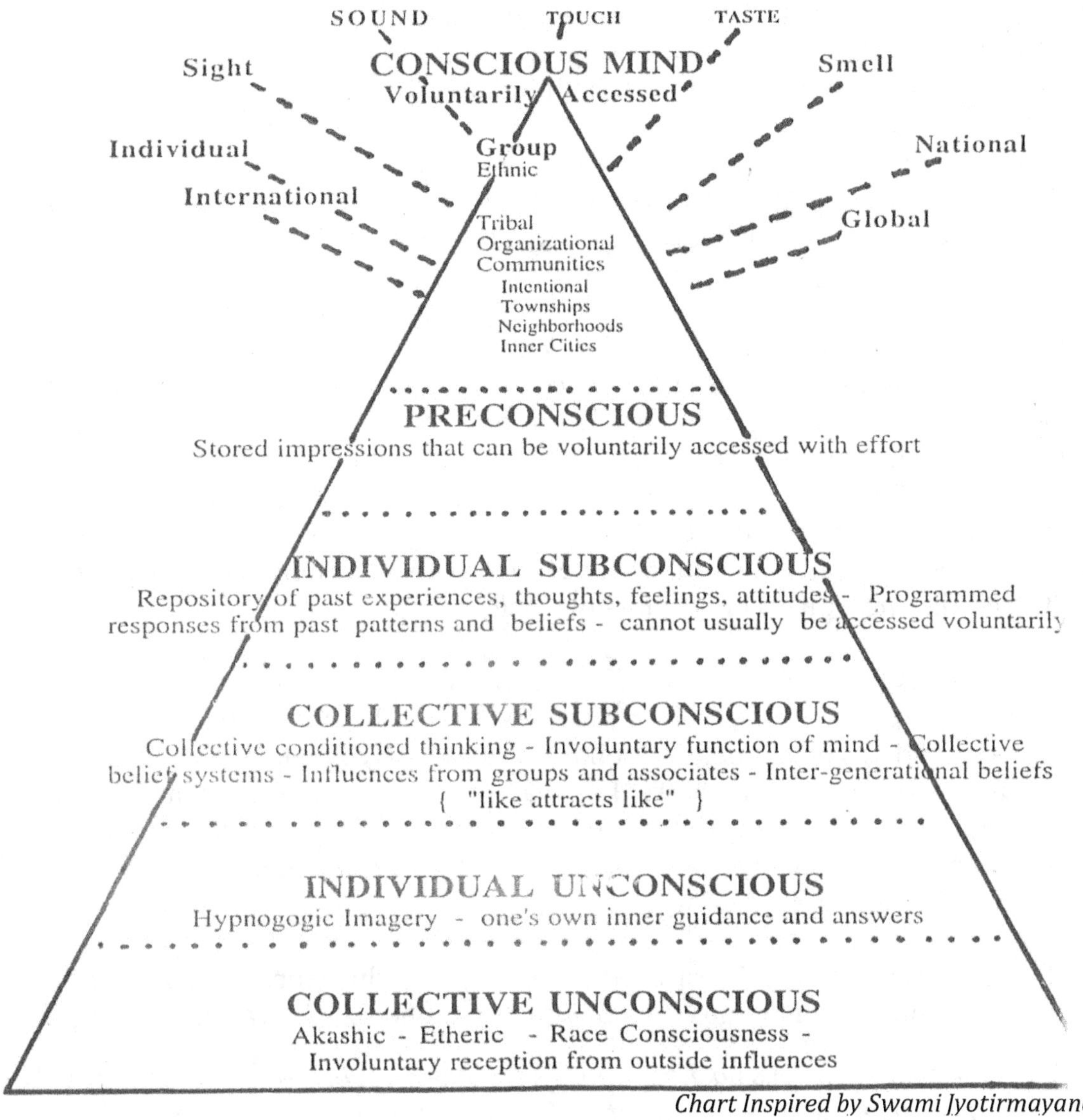

Chart Inspired by Swami Jyotirmayananda

When the subconscious mind is aligned and in harmony with the conscious mind, one is able to manifest their intentions, their visions and dreams. The conscious mind can do a thousand affirmations setting its intentions for what it desires. However, it cannot manifest if the power of the subconscious is not aligned and in agreement with the conscious mind. The conscious mind may be struggling to manifest a better job, home, car and income but lurking in the subconscious vaults of mind may be the thought "I don't deserve it." This would create a conflict between the *manas*, conscious and *citta*, subconscious. This is why affirmations manifest for some and not for others. To manifest there must be alignment between these two states of mind.

The definition of a *yogi* is one who makes the involuntary voluntary. In *haṭha yoga* this might manifest as conscious control of the autonomic nervous system, such as heart beat, respiration and blood pressure. *Yogins* have been known to stop the breath for great lengths of time without dying. Through the breath they can slow down or speed up the heartbeat or even stop the heart.

Being able to make the involuntary voluntary also applies to the mind. The turbulence in the *citta* mind is like the undertow of the ocean. It cannot be seen on the surface but it is an underlying cause of turbulent waves that arise on the surface of the mind.

In making the involuntary voluntary, a *yogin* would be able to remain calm and equanimous throughout life's situations such as praise and blame, fortune and poverty. If one were in touch with the subconscious mind, they would stay centered throughout the hills and valleys of life discerning the origins of impulses (*vṛttis*) that arise from the depth of the *citta*. In seeing the origins of mind waves or *vṛttis* that arise from the subconscious, one can avoid accruing future *karmas* that are the result of desires that lead to action, which gives rise to experiences that result in deposits into the *citta*, the hidden vaults of mind.

The *citta* is the most involuntary part of our being, but by a *yogin*, it can be made to be voluntary. The essence of *yoga* is to hear the thundering hooves of a *vṛtti* or thought wave, and dissolve it before it takes form. As the *yogin* learns to discern the thoughts arising from the *citta* before they manifest, quietness and clarity of mind erases the boundaries between the conscious (*manas*) and subconscious (*citta*). When this happens eventually the *yogin* sees only the divine reflection, realizing oneness with the universal Creator.

When this occurs, the *ahaṁkāra* or ego transmutes into the expression of *buddhi* or over-mind and the *buddhi* merges into *puruṣa*, the timeless substratum of "Being."

***Note**: The manas or conscious part of mind is said to correspond to the front of the body. Citta, the subconscious, which is difficult to see with the physical eye, relates to the back of the body. In the art of sitting for meditation, both the front and back bodies are non-aggressively aligned in finding their center. This would imply bringing the back body, the seat of the subconscious to the front body where the storehouse of hidden impressions can be seen and released. In meditation, if the head is kept in alignment where the center of the brain is balanced over the base of the spine, the mind no longer is in the past or the future, but comes into the present moment. That is meditation.*

> *The invisible must become visible*
> *before it can be eradicated (transformed)"*
>
> *-BKS Iyengar*

AHAṀKĀRA – Ego

Ahaṁ means "I am" and *kāra* from the root verb *kri* means to do or to act. *Ahaṁkāra* literally means, "I am doing" and refers to the ego. Often in life, we identify who we are with what we do in the world. The ego asserts, "I am doing." The *buddhi* mind would say, "It is being done through me."

The *ahaṁkāra* is the part of the mind that takes in sensory stimulus from the *manas.* It sorts, calculates and compares, while remaining in a state of separation. It is the contractive part of the mind that sees differences and immediately begins to compare those differences. It likes one thing and not another. It likes one person and not another. It thinks it has "good" judgment—he's too tall, she's too short, he's too fat, she's too thin. The *ahaṁkāra* loves the word 'too.' It thinks it is the judge, jury and executioner.

The *ahaṁkāra* cannot perceive a unified field of consciousness and continually protects and defends itself from its own annihilation. It is always vigilant, unable to rest, struggling with the polarities of the world. It labors for its own existence and justifies its actions based upon its own survival. It is the preservation of the life force and functional aspect of living in the third dimensional world. But if we remain only in the consciousness of self-preservation, we have difficulty identifying with the larger Self. The larger Self has no need to protect or defend and sees it is in unity with all of humankind.

Actions coming from the *ahaṁkāra* emerge out of effort from the self-will and can lead to over-reaching one's own destiny or dharma. The *ahaṁkāra* sees its actions as coming from itself rather than as a vehicle for divine expression. Hence the definition of *ahaṁkāra* is, "I am doing."

So many of the scriptures of *yoga* refer to the annihilation of the ego. I do not believe in annihilation of the ego, but transformation of the ego into the service of the higher will. We can enlist its energy into the realization of the higher Self.

PERSONAL EGO

In the *ahaṁkāra* or ego mind, we tend towards infatuation, obsession, and identification with things that are temporal and illusory. It acquires money, property and land, claims ownership, and grows attached to items and people. This can lead to suffering when these objects of affection are not available.

The *ahaṁkāra* can envy the qualities in others that it believes to be lacking. Instead of aspiring to greater heights when admiring the gifts, talents, appearances and accomplishments of others, in its forgetfulness of its oneness with all, the *ahaṁkāra* tries to bring the other to the level where it thinks it is, to inflate its own self-worth. In other words, it cuts off the head of another to make itself taller. It may do this through gossip, deprecatory teasing, bullying, cyber-bullying, making fun of others and tearing down their reputation, which is a form of character assassination.

This cute, naughty little *ahaṁkāra* can wreak havoc in our life like a Tasmanian devil. It can stir up everything around it, creating a drama of confusion and imbalance.

Because the ego cannot perceive that there are no 'others,' it competes rather than cooperates. It is the part of the mind that lies and cheats to preserve its own self-interests. In a corporate structure, one may lie to deflect blame by distorting facts of a situation at work. In trying to advance, the ego may try to build its foundation by climbing over the bodies of the competition, destroying reputations in seeking its own self-interests.

Any perspective that is not aligned with the *ahaṁkāra* may threaten it. It believes itself to be 'right' and anyone else who thinks differently is 'wrong.' It sees black and white, right and wrong, justice and injustice. It wants immediate justice or vengeance without the patience of viewing a situation in its entirety.

The *ahaṁkāra* is accelerated through fear; fear of its own annihilation. Fear can cause the *ahaṁkāra* to take rash and forceful action. It may even try to destroy those it perceives as a threat, which can manifest as violent emotions and actions individually and collectively. It thinks and acts defensively causing actions to be on the offensive.

NOTE: There is a difference between ahaṁkāra, ego, & self-esteem. Low self-esteem, as well as overly inflated self-esteem are both an imbalanced conditioned of ahaṁkāra.

GROUP EGO
Mob scenes reflect a group or community ego. In our desire to be part of the group, which is our longing for "Oneness," the *ahaṁkāra* may drive us to transgression of our own integrity. Mob scenes and bullying are examples of the group ego that can infringe on others. It lies to itself to find excuses to invade the territories of others.

NATIONAL EGO
Just as the individual ego can verbally or physically attack an individual, the collective ego of a government can invade the territorial imperative of another country. Under the guise of the military, it feels justified in leaping over boundaries to acquire and occupy countries. It has endless excuses for its questionable actions and territorial greed in the process, numbing itself to the turbulence and pain caused by its actions to the collective sea of humanity.

Because the ego cannot see that there are no 'others,' it needs to have an enemy to justify its own defense system whether individually or collectively. The national ego uses the enemy to arouse fear in the masses, to justify its need to attack another nation. Whether it is personal or national, the ego sees its separated self and fights for its own identity and existence. It cannot perceive a unified field of consciousness.

THE COSMIC JOY OF AHAṀKĀRA

> *Let Us Not Destroy the Ego, Let Us Transform It*

With all that, the *ahaṁkāra* is actually a wonderful aspect for it preserves and protects the life force of the body and nature. The motivating force of self-preservation is powerful. We do not want to destroy it, but to transform it.

It is like a little orphan child that may feel left out and acts out in its need for attention. If we try to push it away we give it more power. Sometimes all it really needs is for us to put our arm around it, reassure it, love it and bring it back into the fold of its universal family.

In identifying with separation, the *ahaṁkāra* cannot see behind and beyond the veil of illusion of separation. The ego can be seen as the humanity within us and as we use the ego to transcend the ego, it transforms itself into the "higher mind" or *buddhi* mind. Eventually the ego gets reabsorbed into the supra-conscious state of *puruṣa* meaning "to fill with the light of the dawn."

Now we will explore different states of the ahaṁkāra as it relates to the three guṇas (For review on the three guṇas, refer to page VIII in the Introduction)

INFERIOR EGO – *Tamasic*

The lethargic ego seems to have a lack of confidence. It is self-conscious, thinking it's never good enough. Fear that relates to the unknown is in every being but the *tamasic* ego does not have the courage to face its fears. It masquerades as humility. It can be passive-aggressive but its nature is to slip into self-blame instead of self-responsibility. It appears humble and passive but due to its fears of confronting an issue or a person directly, it can become aggressive in very subtle ways. Teasing and making fun of others is a passive-aggressive tendency of a *tamasic* ego.

The *tamasic* ego justifies its own existence through quiet and even silent conflict with others. When it is *tamasic,* the ego sees itself as a victim. It wallows in self-pity and even at times, self-blame. This part of ego sees itself as less than others. It gives a feeling of insecurity and inadequacy. It strikes out at others to make itself more important. This false importance can lead to verbal and physical abuse, behind the back gossip, trying to destroy a person's character in the eyes of others. It sabotages itself and others because it doesn't think it's deserving or "good enough." It's absorbed with guilt and anger turning in on itself until guilt and anger become depression and self-punishment.

It sees fear wherever it looks, imagining the worst in any situation. It builds structures to protect and keep others out, not realizing the same structures can lock itself in. To preserve its existence, it represents contraction and constriction, a narrowing of consciousness rather than expansion when faced with a fear. It can numb itself from feeling through its self-chosen addictions. The lethargy of *tamas* can be overcome through *rajas* and eventually *sattva*.

SUPERIOR EGO – *Rajasic*
When the ego is *rajasic,* it strikes out like the tongue of a serpent to blame, criticize and judge others. It sees itself as always right and if others don't agree with its perception, they are wrong. It gravitates towards structure seeking meaning and protection by building fundamentalist belief systems. The *rajasic* ego is restless, clinging to situations that bring momentary pleasure and happiness.

It loves the drama of the hills and valleys of emotions. It surfs the emotional waves sometimes missing a wave and other times paddling too fast. When it gets in front of the wave, the result is emotional "wipe out." This aspect of ego is fearful, which causes a state of chronic tension

The *rajasic* ego imagines itself to be superior to others. It asserts its own strength and is aggressive in its search for self-identity. It is highly competitive, is materially oriented and even spiritually ambitious. It builds edifices of 'self' importance and looks down on others because it can't see its own oneness with others. As a result, it is critical of others because it fears its own loss of position. It busies itself to forget its own non-existence. It clings to life, people and possessions because it fears its own annihilation.

Rajasic ego is self-serving with an "I-me-mine" attitude. Every action is performed for its own self-aggrandizement. It is concerned with its image, looking good to others. It goes to great lengths to protect its own self-image. It has an inflated sense of its own worth. It seeks fame and fortune and serves others only to attain something for itself. It needs adulation and recognition where every action has a self-need embedded in its center. Actions stem out of impure motive such as "what can I get" rather than "what can I give." It's easily angered, impatient and restless. It is harsh in assessment of others and blames others for their faults while seeing itself as 'perfect.' It is easily angered if another criticizes or points out its faults.

Instead of repressing or getting rid of the ego, it can be lovingly coaxed and cajoled, and transformed into Divine service

As the *rajasic* ego becomes more *sattvic*, it can transform into the *buddhi* state of consciousness. *Yoga* is not meant to annihilate the ego but to transform its power into more expansive service of the Divine.

SPIRITUAL EGO – *Sattvic*
This part of ego can be compared with the *sattvic* nature that implies light, lightness and serenity. It hovers beyond the plane of opposites and sees all parts as aspects of the whole. It works with, rather than against the "Higher Self." The *sattvic* or spiritual

ego can feel what others are feeling, holding compassion rather than sympathy. We don't want to deny or repress the ego in any form. The essence of *yoga* is not to annihilate or destroy the ego. The ego gives and preserves life. It maintains and protects the life force. Instead of repressing or getting rid of the ego, it can be lovingly coaxed and cajoled, and transformed into Divine service.

Its energy is powerful as an evolutionary source for transformation of self and in service to the world. Even though it is a contractive part of the mind that produces and feels pain, instead of trying to beat it down, it is important to befriend it, take it into the fold like a long-lost child, and enlist its powerful energy. The power of the ego can be harnessed, transforming it into the service of the *buddhi* mind to become an ally rather than an enemy in the process of transcendence. When the ego is transformed into the light and serenity of *sattva*, it automatically morphs into the *buddhi* consciousness.

The feeling that I am this mortal personality is egoistic while the realization, "I Am The Supreme Self," is the ego-less revelation of the truth of life.

These three states of ego can volley between self-pity and depression projecting outwards in blaming others for its trials and tribulations. It vacillates between repression and self-blame and self-justification for its anger toward others. Eventually it finds its way out of the trap of polarities and begins to refine and rebalance itself. Through practice, it slowly develops the ability to stay balanced amidst all polarities and eventually transmutes itself into the *buddhi* state of consciousness.

We use the ego
to transcend the ego

How Do These Three Parts of Ego Interact With One Another?
It is common for the ego to alternate between *tamas*, *rajas* and *sattva*. At times, it will be calm and serene perceiving all sides of an issue, even when it is being criticized and verbally attacked. It understands the underlying issues of the attack and does not take it personally. Instead, it feels the pain of the other without feeling the need to defend itself or lapsing angrily into blaming the other. It is not repressing but transcending.

At other times, the ego can't quite get above the waves to gain perspective. It lapses into its own pain, not perceiving the origin and when it feels threatened reacts to the symptom of the criticism. It can either become *rajasic*, hurling anger and criticism back at its source and going on the attack itself, or it lapses into a *tamasic* mode of shock feeling sorry for itself, holding the anger within, thereby creating future illness of the body or depression that comes through continual repression of emotion. In this state, the mind continues to replay the situation, dramatically building upon it by having imaginary conversations of what it should have said and plotting its vindication or even revenge at some later time. It cannot quite gather its courage to face the situation directly so it cowers in a mental corner waiting for its opportunity to strike out. Sometimes the strike is projected onto another that happens to do or say something that triggers a memory of an event that has nothing to do with the original situation. "Where did *that* come from?" is the usual response.

The ego may fluctuate and alternate between these three phases. Continual practice and self-observation weakens the downward pull of the ego and eventually we can offer it up to the *buddhi* (like a sacrificial offering) for its own transformation.

BUDDHI - Intellect or Over-mind

Bodh means *To Know*

The development of the buddhi mind is the sacred task of every yoga aspirant

The over-mind or intellect is the part of mind that reasons, analyzes, asserts and arranges. It is not to be confused with intellection, the process of understanding. All creativity stems from the development of intellect. It is this intellect that blooms into intuition revealing the mystic self—the universal consciousness. Therefore, all philosophical developments pursue the path of reason and culminate in the intuitive realization where reason is fulfilled and transcended. Intellect balances and integrates reason and feeling. In the *buddhi* states of mind, there are no separative polarities such as likes and dislikes. It holds the bigger picture through discrimination, seeing differences but not comparing them.

The *buddhi* mind has the ability to hold two or more points of perspective simultaneously without making one wrong and the other right. It is a state of "choice-less awareness." When we are in the *buddhi* state of mind, it is as if we were standing on a mountaintop with 360-degree unobstructed view. This state of mind does not dwell in the separative contractive self, but is expansive in its ability to embrace all beings within the light of its consciousness.

It is this over-mind of *buddhi* that transforms intellect into intuition. Intuition is the mystic gate to liberation that is latent within every individual. The intellect is actually a conditioned aspect of intuition. It studies the world in fragments and can only bring us a tiny fragment of the cosmic whole. It keeps us bound in what we perceive as "reality."

In Vedānta, intuition is known as *brahmakāra vṛtti.* This means that the mind has developed a profound insight into the illusion of objects by understanding that God or *Brahman* is the reality behind everything. It is said that the truly intuitive mind flows only toward *Brahman*. Its only ruling thought is of the creator. If we want to develop intuition and dwell in the *buddhi* state of mind, it is recommended that we keep the mind from continually shifting from the past to the future and back to the past. In the *buddhi* state, the mind gracefully stays in the moment regardless of what we are doing or not doing. The development of the *buddhi* mind is the sacred task of every *yoga* aspirant.

> *All philosophical developments pursue the path of reason and culminate in the intuitive realization where reason is fulfilled and transcended*

The *buddhi* is a powerful onlooker, a witness, and the non-doer. It is the nucleus of what the *Bhagavad Gītā* mentions as the "inaction within the action." It is able to see behind the surface of a situation perceiving cause and not just affect. It does not judge, criticize or condemn but holds the balance between all polarities such as justice and injustice, compliment and criticism, praise and blame, good and not so good, light and dark.

Instead of being 'wishy-washy,' the *buddhi* consciousness is a powerful state of 'Being.' It acts but does not react. It does not have an attachment to a result. The actions that stem from the *buddhi* are so powerful that they don't just change a situation but transform it for the betterment of all. It is not sympathetic but is compassionate for all beings, understanding the nature of suffering and transcending it at the same time. It holds to the remembrance of a place beyond the "sea of *saṃsāra*," pain and suffering on a human plane. In consciousness, it is able to touch the hem of the garment of the great ones existing on a plane invisible to the 3rd dimensional eye.

When we are in the 'over-mind' or *buddhi* consciousness, it is easier to relate in interactions with others, especially family members. In this state of mind, we have no expectations and are not trying to mold others into our concept of perfection. Even critical words or thoughts won't carry the sting and pains of the past. Because we can see the deeper issues that contributed to projected judgment and condemnations of the past, we don't take it on, even if it is meant to be personal. We don't even blame or judge others for having judged.

The Dalai Lama once gave an equation for the definition of compassion, "Love plus detachment equals compassion." When we can uncover the place of deepest compassion within our being, there is no superiority. We embrace all as the brothers and sisters of the one humanity, understanding the nature of those who may strike out at us or others, and addressing situations clearly and decisively without blame or expectation of a result.

In the *buddhi* state the ego surrenders itself in service of the Divine and the light of God, like the sun, radiates from the core of our being. In this non-judgmental state,

our environment and all who dwell within it cannot adversely influence us. We grow stronger.
An individual who holds the *buddhi* consciousness is like a giant tree that spread its branches in all directions. All those who come under its umbrella are given shade and protection. It does not withdraw its branches from some while giving to others

The *buddhi* consciousness is like the sun casting its rays in every direction giving light to all equally. It is equanimous, serene, compassionate and expansive. It does not create waves or ripples that have negative or positive repercussions of *karma* whether in this life or beyond. The *buddhi* mind shines as the reflection of *puruṣa*, the undifferentiated timeless state of being.

Intuitional enlightenment of the *buddhi* mind will not affect the practical realities of our lives, but it is like a magic wand. It gives new meaning, new significance and a new dimension to everything that we touch, everything that we do.

THE CHARIOT AND FOUR PARTS OF MIND

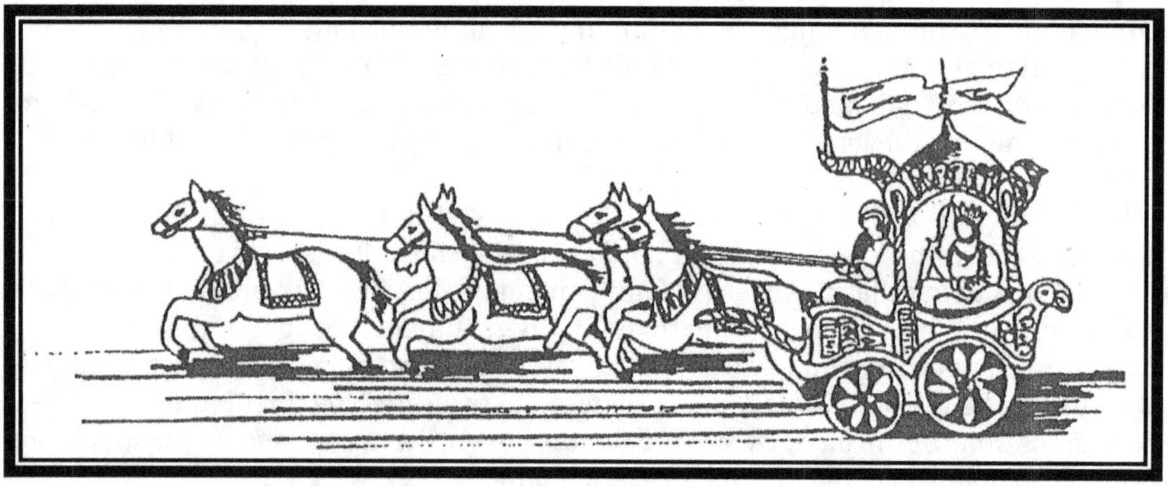

Swami Jyotirmayānanda, a direct disciple of Master Sivānanda, uses an allegory from the *Kaṭha Upaniṣads* to describe the way the four parts of mind work together that relate to a chariot and the five horses traveling over the roads of life.

The chariot is the body and the rider is the *Ātman* or individual soul. The five horses represent the five senses and the reins are the *manas*, the conscious mind. The reins of *manas* control the five senses and are in the hands of the driver that can be either the *buddhi* or the *ahaṁkāra*.

Four Parts of Mind

Conscious

Sensory perceptions...action oriented. Takes in sights, sounds, smells, taste and touch of the outer world... mental/thinking...cognitive processes

Overmind

Overview - Intuitive part of mind... where intellect is transformed into higher intuition. Sees differences and variances but does not compare those differences. Choicelessly aware, with focused mind that can hold two or more points of view simultaneously.

Ego

Places value on sensory perception... protects, defends... is territorial... fearful, sees separation. Compares differences: "I like that... I don't like that..."

Subconscious

Storehouse of conscious impressions. "Every conscious experience becomes a subconscious impression." Before real change can occur when one's thinking, actions and life... must first overhaul subconscious. Several layers.

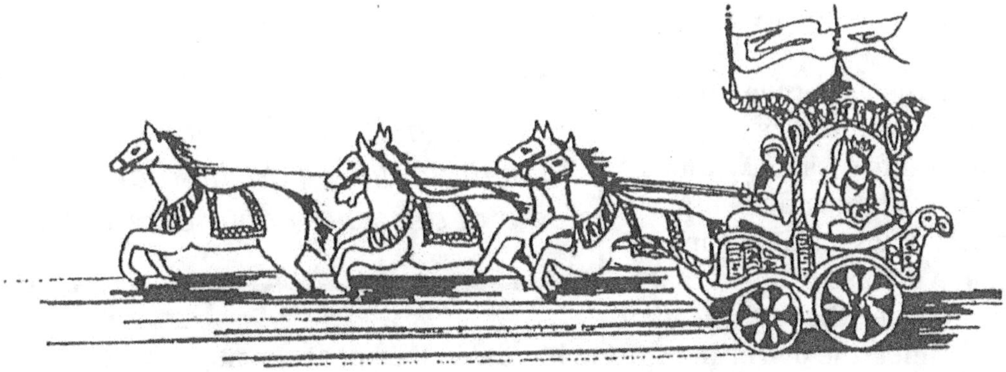

The chariot, horses, driver and rider are travelling over the roads of life's polarities such as virtue and vice, light and dark, expansion and contraction, hills and valleys toward the destination of self-realization or self-actualization. Their arrival at the destination is determined by which part of the mind is in the driver's seat. Is it the *buddhi*, the over-mind, or is it the *ahaṁkāra*, the ego that is holding the reins? If the reins are in the hands of the *ahaṁkāra*, the chariot may be deflected from the original goal or intention. It may be blown by the winds of desire and lack of focus and in confusion, wander circuitously losing sight of the intended goal. As it loses its way, it travels over rocky and difficult paths of life's polarities that may threaten to overturn or destroy the chariot that is the vehicle of the Soul. If the *ahaṁkāra* loses control of the reins, the horses can scatter creating a delay or premature end to the journey.

If the horses, which symbolize the five senses, do not feel the control of the reins of *manas*, the conscious mind, they may lack direction and become confused. This can take the chariot of the body and the rider of the *Ātman*, the individual soul over difficult terrain, even over a cliff. The chariot may be destroyed and the horses of the senses scattered. Other times, the journey may end in a cul-de-sac, moving away from the goal but eventually leading back to the original path.

However, if the reins of the horses are in the hands of the *buddhi* mind, the chariot will be brought directly to its self-realized destination. To do this, the driver requires:

- Perseverance
- Patience
- Non-attachment
- Devotion
- Dedication
- Discrimination
- Sincerity and truthfulness
- Sensitivity and compassion

To bring the chariot, the horses and the rider to a successful destination, the driver must be compassionate, intuitive and sensitive to Divine guidance.

> *The buddhi mind can give wisdom, insight and compassion that are born out of the ashes of our own suffering*

In *buddhi*, the driver would be non-critical seeing all sides of the road or life's issues without judging one right and the other wrong. At times, he or she may travel in a light so brilliant that they cannot see the way ahead. At other times, the driver may grope blindly in darkness sensing, not seeing and having to slowly guide the movement of the horses and the chariot with faith.

The driver requires clear vision and right discrimination when traveling the road through the center of darkness and light, life's joys and sorrows. At times, there will be the crossing of the bridges of tears and laughter, through the valleys of sacrifice to the mountaintops of unobstructed vision and understanding.

At times, life's emotional crises require decisive action; at other times, it can take the form of a great and vital test. There may be a brief period of time that calls forth every resource of strength, wisdom, clarity of purpose and purity of motive that we may possess. If life's crises continue, over a long period of time producing emotional strain which carries over onto many years of living, this can create mental strain and eventually filter into the body which may carry the burden then of ill health and physical ailments. The *buddhi* mind can give wisdom, insight and compassion that are born out of the ashes of our own suffering. If we don't recognize the guidance in a subtle form, we will be given it in a not so subtle and more recognizable form. In other words, if we do not feel the touch of a feather, we may be hit on the head with a hammer.

Another similar analogy can be found in the *Bhagavad Gītā*, the sixth canto of the *Mahābhārata*. As the two armies of the *Kauravas* and *Pandavas*, the dark and light forces are poised on opposite ends of the battlefield of *Kurukśetra* waiting for the call to begin the battle. There is great significance in this image. The Sanskrit word *kuru* means moving from darkness to light and *kśetra* means destroying in order to transcend. So, in the field where the forces of polarities are intended to meet, it is the field where the warriors move from "darkness to light, destroying in order to transcend." The *Kauravas*, opposing forces of the *Pandavas*, represent darkness, or the egoistic contraction that can only see and care about its own agenda. The *Pandavas* or light forces represent the warriors that are about to destroy or transform the ego, in order for transcendence for all, merging into the same light of Divinity in the remembrance that we are already one with the universal source of being.

Here too, the individual soul enters onto the field of *Kurukśetra*, holding the remembrance of non-attachment to a result or even the desire to win. To emerge unscathed from the battle requires perseverance, patience, devotion, dedication and discrimination. It also requires sensitivity, compassion, integrity and concentration. As the Bible says, "If thine eye be single, thy whole body will be filled with light."

The field of *Kurukśetra* exists on the subtle or astral plane. It is the field of life's polarities, like the road with the chariot. The field is humanity as a whole and the individual human unity. The individual soul (the warrior) prepares itself to enter into the battle of the transformation of the ego. It is a wonderful analogy as we go about the daily routine of life, observing if we are in the ego part of our mind or in the *buddhi* mind. This field is the razor's edge of polarities that can seduce us from one side to the other. The intent is to remain unattached to either polarity and stay centered in the midst of the turbulence of life's joys and crises. This analogy is the ultimate in non-attachment, even the non-attachment to a result. This is the true *karma yoga*.

YOGAŚ CITTA VṚTTI NIRODAḤ IN ĀSANA

This *sūtra* can be practiced in every *āsana*.

Traditionally it was believed that *āsana* was practiced to curb the restlessness of the body in order to make the mind fit for meditation. Why wait? Patañjali says there is only one *āsana* — *dhyānāsana*, the pose of meditation. The seat of meditation can be found within the center of every *āsana*. The breath within *āsana* acts as a barometer reflecting varying states of mind and emotions while in the pose (see breath and the five states of mind in *prāṇāyāma*, II:50).

Commentaries on the *sūtras* say *prāṇāyāma* practiced with a restless mind produces more restlessness. I have found that *āsana* practiced without breath produces a restless mind. The essence of all *yoga* is to quiet the turbulence of the waves of the mind. To do this, it is essential to use the breath in *āsana*.

> *The seat of meditation can be found within the center of every Āsana*

The breath will reflect the varying states of mind and can be experienced as a gauge as to the calmness or turbulence of the mind. When the mind waves become still like a placid lake, we can see our own reflection and realize we are already one with the universal source. It is the turbulence and distortion of the waves that arise and fall in the mind that keep us from seeing and knowing this. There are times in *āsana*, when the breath and the mind become effortlessly still. The pose then becomes a pose of meditation (*dhyāna*) and if sustained can lead to the first stages of *samādhi*. This point of stillness, or *bindu*, can be found in the practice of *āsana*. The *bindu* is the seed of each *āsana* out of which the pose emerges and returns.

To find stillness of mind in the action of *āsana*, it is helpful to begin in simple poses and slowly graduate to more complex. You can start in *Mārjāryāsana* (cat stretch) and once the breathing and elongation is mastered observe if the same rhythm of breath and quietness of mind can be maintained when bringing the buttock up into *Adho Mukha Śvānāsana* (downward facing dog).

Did you maintain the same rhythm of the breath? A quiet mind will be revealed in the breath as well as relaxation of head, neck and face. Once the breath in this pose is mastered, can you bring one leg up into *Eka Pada Adho Mukha Śvānāsana* (one-legged downward facing dog)? If the breath becomes labored and erratic, use a support for the upper leg (such as a wall), and practice calming the breath and in turn, the mind within the pose without losing the elongation of the lift. If the breath is still erratic, shallow and rapid, come out of the pose. Regain a calm breath in the cat stretch or the child's pose. Try again or wait for another day.

If practicing preparation for headstand, observe the breath because it reflects either a tranquil or turbulent mind. Is it telling you that you can walk the legs a little further toward the torso or stop at a given point to regain its calmness? Are you breathing while lifting the buttock bones to the sky as the forearms and bottom wrist bone press into the earth? As you walk in, does the breath change? Is it possible for you to wait on that edge before proceeding further? Can you wait until a calm breath reflecting a calm mind tells you it's okay to proceed? Can you maintain the breath when lifting one leg on the exhalation? Can you maintain the same rhythmic breath when lifting the opposite leg?

To practice this *sūtra* within *āsana*, we can evaluate: have we stopped breathing, are we holding tension in our neck and face in trying "to get" the pose? Are we trying to rush breathlessly into the next phase of the pose or are we enjoying the beauty of the journey as well as the destination? If we move into *āsana* on the exhalation rather than the inhalation, the mind has an opportunity to remain in a tranquil state during the action of the pose. If we stop at each interval during the inhalation and do nothing, something magical happens. In breathing in this way during *āsana*, the pose can bring the mind effortlessly into the state of *Yogaś Citta Vṛtti Nirodhaḥ*.

> *"Sūtras weave within a posture like a thread – like a string of pearls. The sūtra thread binds us, woven to a central theme, awareness of Self. Every part of the body is like a pearl, every part wedded to the Self"*
>
> *-BKS Iyengar*

EXERCISE:

Discuss or Journal on the Following Questions:

1) *Name the Four Parts of Mind, in Sanskrit and English.*
2) *Which part of mind do you feel is in the driver's seat of your life? Why?*
3) *Which aspect of the mind do you tend toward when faced with life's challenges? Please explain.*
4) *Can you identify some patterns and beliefs that originate from the citta, subconscious layers of mind, and affected your behaviors in life? Please describe.*
5) *Describe your understanding of ahaṁkāra, ego mind. How can ahaṁkāra be beneficial? How do you see your ahaṁkāra in relation to the three guṇas, is it tamasic, rajasic or sattvic?*
6) *Give an example from your life, when you have been able to view a situation from buddhi mind.*
7) *How do the Four Parts of Mind relate to your āsana practice?*

HOMEPLAY: *Take one week to one month and observe the interaction of these four parts of mind in your daily life. Keep a daily journal if possible, as it will be invaluable in weaving the Sūtras into your life.*

I.3 TADĀ DRAṢṬUḤ SVARŪPE AVASTĀNAM

Tadā *= Then*
Draṣṭuḥ *= the seer*
Sva *= one's own*
Rūpe (Rupa) *= form*
Ava *= coming down near*
Stā *= establish*
Nam *= to revere*

This third *sūtra* could be literally translated as:
(When The Waves Of The Mind Are Still) Then The Seer Comes Down Near And Establishes Itself (With Reverence) Within Its Own Form.

Translations are usually:
Then The Seer Abides In Itself.
Then The Seer (Self) Abides In Its Own Nature.
The Seer And Seen Abide In His Own Form.

I translate this as:
The Seer And Seen Become One OR Realize The Oneness (Union) That Already Is.

If we believe that the union of *yoga* already exists and all the practices we do is to unfold into the experience of that union or oneness, then we could more accurately interpret this *sūtra* as: Realize the oneness that already is.

This *sūtra* is the end of the game. There is no need to go any further. This is the state of oneness, *kaivalya*, liberation, and '*Citta Vṛtti Nirodaḥ*,' where the waves of the mind are so still that the realization dawns of that which already is.

This *sūtra* gives the ultimate essence of why we are practicing *yoga*. Here, Patañjali describes what happens when the waves (*vṛttis*) of the mind (*citta*) are quiet and still and no longer turbulent. The term suppression is usually used to describe this state of stillness of the waves of the mind. I find that our intent here is not to repress or suppress the waves but to bring them to a state of balanced quiescence and divine stillness.

When this happens, the mind waves then become so still, like the waters of a lake on a windless day. As we gaze into its depths, we see only our own reflection. This is the state when the seer and the seen become one—or realize the oneness that already is. We could not see that union before because when the waves of the waters of the mind were turbulent, it could not radiate the Divine reflection that is our own.

> *"Go From What You See To What Sees"*
>
> *-Sir T.K.V. Desikachar*

When the *sūtra* speaks of the "seer" and the "seen" it is interesting to note that the *buddhi*, the knower, is considered to be the seen and *puruṣa,* meaning to fill with the dawn, is the seer. Ancient sages say that the *buddhi* or the I-sense that is the instrument of knowledge cannot even illumine its own self. It shines from the reflection of *puruṣa* that is the vehicle through which all actions of *buddhi* are manifested. *Puruṣa* is known as "pure consciousness." When pure consciousness, the seer, abides in its own self as it does in the state of liberation, we can then know and experience the union of *puruṣa* as the seer, the impartial witness, and *buddhi*, the seen.

The word *draṣṭuḥ* relates to *puruṣa* and means perceiving. Sir Desikachar once said in a *sūtra* class in India, "Some schools see the mind as a sense." Then he asked, "In *draṣṭuḥ*, are we perceiving, the mind...or what is behind the mind?" I wondered, "Would this then be the seer? If we were to perceive what is behind the mind, would we then have the experience of *puruṣa*, the seer?

As if reading my thoughts, Sir Desikachar answered, "*Draṣṭuḥ* is the source of life that draws other things into its field of awareness. *Draṣṭuḥ* is *puruṣa*! It is the constant observer. In sleep for instance, something is not sleeping." What is that which is ever awake? *Draṣṭuḥ* can be seen as the illumination of the sun. The light of the sun comes into the mind and illumines it but it is not the mind. Without *draṣṭuḥ*, the mind cannot function.

"The person in a state of *yoga* is not connected to anything outside, only to what is already within," Sir Desikachar seemed for a moment to ponder his own statement and then spontaneously said, "We know about the things outside of ourselves but so little about ourselves." He then went on to say that the human structure is not just the body. "In *yoga*, it starts with body and then we move from the gross to the subtle." It is as if Patañjali is saying, "go from what you see to what sees." I translated this as what Mr. B.K.S. Iyengar would say, "moving from the known to the unknown."

This *sūtra* is a little difficult to understand in the very beginning of the book. This is why there are so many more *sūtras* to explain and give instructions as to how we can experience the state of consciousness where the seer and the seen become one.

> *Draṣṭuḥ can be seen as the illumination of the sun. The light of the sun comes into the mind and illumines it but it is not the mind. Without driṣṭa, the mind cannot function.*

IN ĀSANA

In *āsana*, we can experience this sense of becoming one with the source if the pose is done as an offering of one's self to the universal until eventually, the gap of separation closes as the waves of the mind grow calm and still. This will reflect in the closing of the gap between the inhalation and exhalation. When the two breaths merge into one another in the *āsana*, the breath appears to have stopped. This state is the essence of all *prāṇāyāma* practices known as *kevala kumbhaka*, which means the retention of that which is isolated and absolutely pure. It is as if we are not breathing—but breath IS. In this state in the *āsana*, the mind becomes so quiet and calm that it draws consciousness into itself (*pratyāhāra*) and then in an instant the mind becomes one pointed (*dhāraṇā*) and then merges into a sense of wholeness or oneness where subject and object merge (*dhyāna*). If this retention of mind and breath are held for as little as 12 seconds our consciousness enters the first stage of *samādhi*. *Samādhi* is the state where "the seer and seen abide in his/her own form." It is not something that is beyond our reach and unattainable. It is as close as our own breath and can happen spontaneously within any *āsana*. This is why it is important in the practice of *āsana* to allow the breath to move the body into the pose.

I.4 VṚTTI SĀRŪPYAM ITARATRA

Vṛtti = *waves of the mind*
Sa = *with*
Rūpa = *form*
Ita = *like*
Ratra = *the night*

The Vṛttis, Or Mind Waves, Are With Or Take The Form (Like) Of The Night.

Translations are usually:
At Other Times, The Seer Appears To Assume The Modifications Of The Mind.
At Other Times, (The Self Appears To) Assume The Forms Of The Mental Modifications.

In this particular *sūtra*, I prefer the translation from my Sanskrit teacher, "The *vṛttis* take the form of the night." It seems more accurate and more interesting. Here we see Patañjali lyrically modulating from one *sūtra* to the next. The previous *sūtra* seems so final and complete in fulfilling the tenants of *yoga*. Basically, he is giving away the plot by saying, "When the waves of the mind are still, the seer and the seen become one." We may as well close our book and read no further. However, in this fourth *sūtra* Patañjali tells why we should continue.

It's as if the author seems to be saying something like, "But, this is not an easy task to quiet the waves of the mind and for the seer to abide in its own form"—BECAUSE—the *vṛttis* take the form of the unseen which is like the night. We cannot see them. They are lying in the depths of the subconscious mind. We cannot easily access them as they are considered to be involuntary."

Yoga practices are meant to bring the involuntary to the level of the voluntary, or the subconscious impressions to the level of the conscious mind where they can be seen and, in turn, transformed.

The mind waves that arise from the unseen depths of the psyche are powerful motivators, propelling us to say or do things that can result in positive or negative experiences. These experiences would then create impressions in varying layers of our subconscious psyche. There is a saying in *yoga*, that "every conscious experience becomes a subconscious impression." These impressions are known as *saṃskāras*. Eventually, the *saṃskāras* emerge as a new *vṛtti*. The *vṛttis* are the mental modifications of the mind that arise out of the depth of our subconscious as painful or non-painful or a mixture of both. Now, we will discuss the *vṛttis* in more detail.

I.5 VṚTTAYAḤ PAÑCATAYYAḤ KLIṢṬĀKLIṢṬĀḤ

Vṛttayaḥ *= refers to the vṛttis (mind waves)*
Pañcatayyaḥ *= five-fold*
Kliṣṭaḥ *= painful*
Akliṣṭaḥ *= non-painful*

The *Vṛttis* Are Five-Fold, Painful And Non-Painful.

VṚTTIS

Vṛ means to rise upwards or come into existence. *Vṛttis* are sometimes defined as electrical impulses that arise within the field of the mind (*citta*). These impulses lead to a desire and the desire to an action. Out of action comes an experience (either painful or non-painful) and that experience leads to an impression in the psyche. Impressions known as *saṃskāras* are then the reason for the next *vṛtti* to arise. This is called the "Wheel of Cause and Affect" (see II:12). It is a never-ending cycle, the scriptures say, not just in this life, but lives to come.

The mind waves of the *vṛttis* are classified in this *sūtra* as five painful and five non-painful. Patañjali expounds upon the five non-painful mind waves in the following *sūtras* in this chapter. He doesn't mention the five painful *vṛttis* until chapter II. The five painful *vṛttis* are the reason for our afflictions and pain in life. They are called *kleśas* meaning to inflict or afflict. He gives the method of their eradication in Chapter II and III as *aṣṭaṅga yoga*, the eight-fold path or the "Eight Limbs of *Yoga*."

Patañjali seems to build upon the second *sūtra* alluding to the essence of *yoga*, which is to "quiet or still the waves that arise in the field of the mind (*citta*)." Depending upon which part of the field of mind is operative (a*haṁkāra* or *buddhi*) will determine the experience and the way in which impressions are deposited in the psyche. As he says here, these mind waves can be either painful or non-painful.

It should be noted that throughout the *sūtras*, Patañjali does not address emotions, but instead he outlines the source of emotions, which are the way in which the *vṛttis* interact with one another. In Latin, the prefix 'e' means to project outward and *motare* means motion. Therefore, the word emotion would mean to project motion outwards. Emotion has also been defined as "to move away from." This could imply that in emotion we move away from ourselves, or the 'center' of Self.

We can't control the world around us
if we can't control our own minds

Motive and emotion relate to one another. Our motive is what moves us. An example of this would be, "If I love someone, I want them to love me back." Our actions may be motivated out of a desire for love, approval, recognition, appreciation, money, power or pleasing a parent for fear of punishment. I may want to be kind to you, because I want you to be kind to me. When the needs of the ego become involved in the following mind waves, the non-painful *vṛttis* can become painful.

EXERCISE:

Non-painful vṛttis and painful vṛttis (kleśas) are the origin as well as the effects of emotions. We find in the Yoga Sūtras that emotion is the effect, not the cause of turbulent thought waves of the mind. The sūtras address cause as well as effect.

Discuss or Journal on the Following Questions:

1) *What part of the mind causes the non-painful vṛttis to become painful?*
2) *If emotions are the effect of the interaction of the vṛttis, what is the cause of the emotions? Please give an example.*

THE POWER OF THOUGHT WAVES (VṚTTIS)

Yoga scriptures relate the mind to a monkey—not just an ordinary monkey but a drunken money—and not just a drunken monkey but a drunken monkey that has been bitten by a scorpion!

Every thought wave that is projected from a center of consciousness sets up thought wave vibrations. Vibrations from a force field in the surrounding aura create certain patterns. The vibrating thought field proceeds to attract into its "galaxy" atoms of a similar nature. Thoughts are contagious. If we hold a thought and continually repeat it, others will begin to act out the nature of our thought.

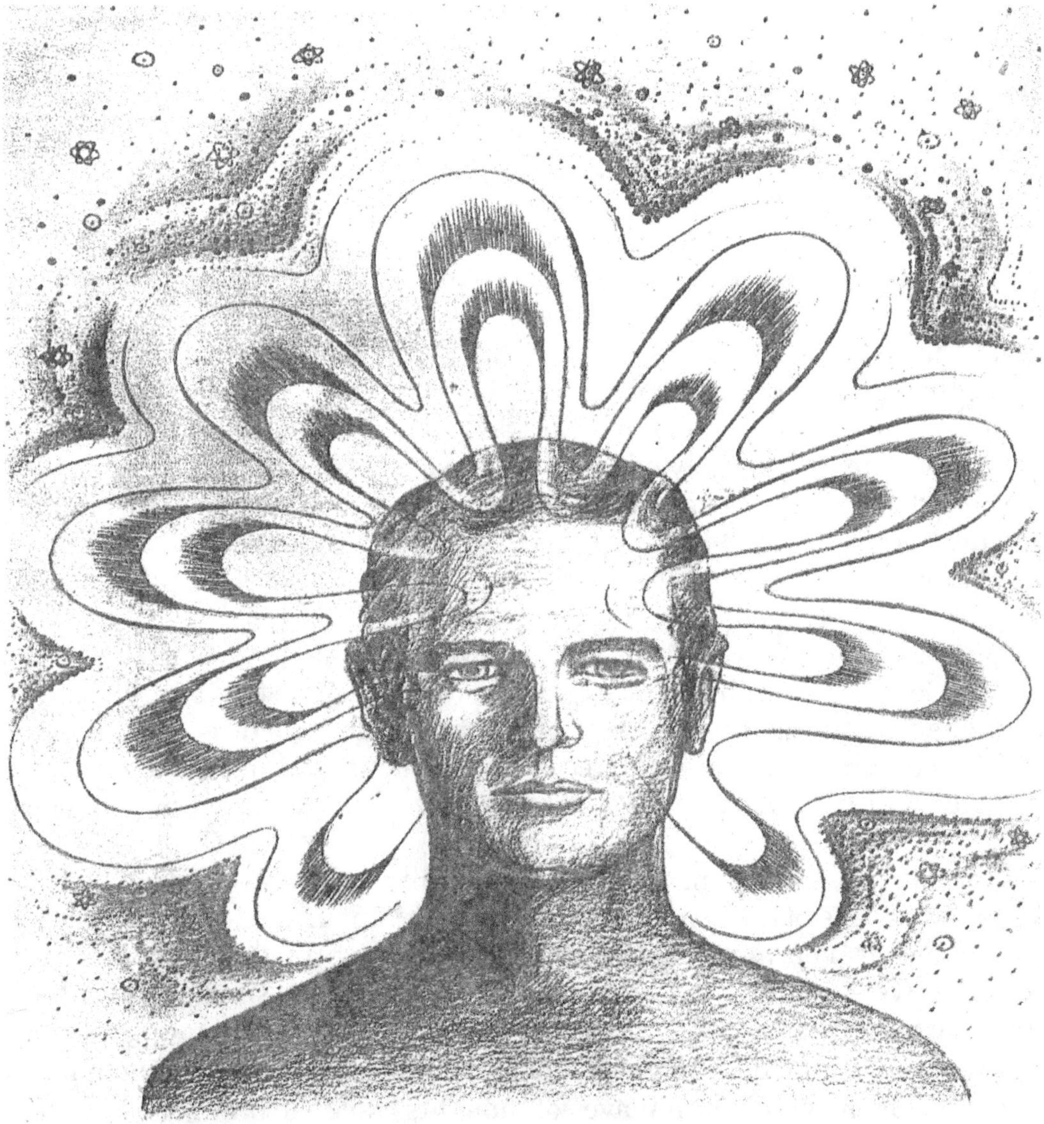

THINKING TRUE

"Every thought wave that is projected from a center of consciousness sets up thought wave vibrations. The vibration from a force field in the surrounding aura creates certain patterns. The vibrating thought field proceeds to attract into its 'galaxy' atoms of a similar nature."

Helena Roerick in her book *Heart* writes, "Disorderly thoughts are contagious. They injure the subtle substance of our 'being' as well as that of others. These thoughts radiate outward to a distance that reflects the intensity of the thought."

Swami Śivānanda of Rishikesh writes that it is important to avoid thoughts of another person's defects. He says, "The nature of the mind is such that it becomes that which it intensely thinks of. Thus, if you think of the vices and defects of another, your mind will be charged with these vices and defects. One who knows this psychological law will never indulge in censuring or in finding fault in the conduct or actions of others. They will only see and praise the good in others. This practice enables one to grow in concentration, *yoga* and spirituality."

Based upon ancient scriptural knowledge as well as experience, Swamiji warns, "Be careful of your thoughts. Whatever you send out of your mind comes back to you. Every thought you think is a boomerang. If you hate another, hate will come back to you. If you love others, love will come back to you. An evil thought is thrice cursed. First, it harms the thinker by doing injury to his/her mental body. Secondly, it harms the person who is its object. Lastly, it harms all mankind by vitiating the whole mental atmosphere."

Our thoughts create a powerful energetic force field. Thought dynamics are influencing not just our own lives, they are also impacting our planetary and universal environment. We may desire world peace but cannot find peace within our own heart and mind. We may want to end the violence and chaos around us but cannot contribute because of the violent and angry thoughts, confusion and chaos within our own mental atmosphere.

Master Śivānanda wrote extensively on the power of thought. "When a thought of good or evil leaves the brain and hovers about it, it gives rise to vibrations in the *manas* or mental atmosphere, which travel far and wide in all directions. It enters the brains of others also. Those who try to purify themselves in a cave or in the marketplace are uplifting humanity and all living creatures throughout the world.

"Just as the sun goes on continuously converting into vapour every drop of water that is on the surface of the earth and just as all the vapour thus rising up gathers together in the form of clouds, all the thoughts that you project from your own lonely corner will mount up and be wafted across space, join similar thoughts projected by those who are like you and, in the end, all these holy thoughts will come down with tremendous force to subjugate undesirable forces. Thoughts are more contagious than influenza. Waves of thoughts leave the brain of one person and enter the brain of another (regardless of distance). A thought of anger produces a similar vibration in those who surround an angry man. A cheerful thought produces cheerful thoughts in others. A thought of joy in us creates sympathetically a thought of joy in others. Carry any kind of thought with you and as long as you retain it, wherever you go, whatever you do, it will attract to yourself those things which correspond to the quality of that thought."

It is reiterated in a variety of ways in Eastern scriptures that the last thought will govern one's future destiny. In other words, the last thought determines the next birth. It is said that Mahatma Gandhi's last word that reflected a lifetime of thought was "Ram," a name of God. It was his life's mantra. It is believed that the last thought is not independent. Rather, it is a compendium of conscious and subconscious thoughts we have gathered throughout our lives. The last prominent thought of one's life occupies the mind at the time of death. The last thought determines the nature of character of the body to be attained next. "As a man thinketh, so shall he become," this biblical theme has continued in the teachings throughout the centuries. Dale Carnegie said in a variety of ways, "Thoughts held in mind produce after their kind."

The *Yoga Sūtras* give us a living, breathing map of how we can transform and subdue (not repress) the thought waves of our mind to transform our lives and realize that we are the fashioners of miracles and the arcitects of our own destiny.

NOTE: THOUGHTS AND DNA
Our thoughts can create physical and chemical structure of a DNA molecule. This is linked to the connection of angry thoughts to cancerous tissue growth. We can wind the DNA at a distance, which will affect the DNA quantitatively across the world. That is the source field of citta. When asked if love has a direct affect on the DNA, scientists have said that love can be seen as a basic principle of universal energy. The DNA spiral can be seen as the kundalini. DNA is a wave structure that can be rearranged. We can rewrite our own DNA to adapt to nature. The source field, related to citta, appears in the DNA as virtual photons that are stored for useable energy.

I.6 PRAMĀṆA VIPARYAYA VIKALPA NIDRĀ SMṚTAYAḤ

***Pramāṇa** = from prā to bring forth and mana from manas, the mind. Pramāṇa is correct or accurate perceptions.*
***Viparyaya** = Vi means to reverse or negate and par to fill or to perceive and yaya gives it force. This would then mean REALLY not seeing or perceiving. Viparyaya is inaccurate or incorrect perception*
***Vikalpa** – Vi negates or reverses and kalpa is time. This word literally means no time. It is translated as imagination.*
***Nidrā** = sleep (physical and psychological)*
***Smṛti** = memory, from sma, to remember*

The Non-Painful Vṛttis Are Correct Perception, Incorrect Perception, Imagination, Sleep And Memory.

The non-painful *vṛttis* are given in the next few versus and the painful mind waves are given in the second chapter as the *kleśas* (the reason for our afflictions in life). Even the non-painful *vṛttis* however, can become painful if the ego mind becomes involved. When the *buddhi* mind is in the driver's seat, then the following five mind waves would be non-painful.

FIVE NON-PAINFUL MIND WAVES

The five non-painful mind waves known as *vṛttis*, are:

1) *Pramāṇa*: Correct Perception

This function reveals the reality of things. The three types of perception are direct, indirect and inference. Perception comes from what is already stored in the mind. The mind, in *pramāṇa*, can always be changed. When we change the mind through the practices of *yoga*, our perception changes.

2) *Viparyaya*: Incorrect Perception

This is faulty perception or misconception based upon facts. Often related to a snake being mistaken for a rope in semi-darkness, which causes fear.

3) *Vikalpa*: Imagination

This is imagining due to no underlying reality, different than wrongly perceiving something based upon reality. In imagination, we can distort perceptions based upon no facts and create something out of nothing. This is where we find images that we project onto others and that which gets projected onto us.

4) *Nidrā*: Sleep

This is the function where *citta* (mind-stuff) internalizes itself, withdrawing its energy from physical organs making them 'unconscious' along with the subtle senses and conscious mind. In sleep, there is a total absence of experience and all mental functions. This is a process of the unconscious, which makes us ignore an experience to turn away from a present fact, to 'sleep' in a certain situation. There are three types of sleep, physical, psychological and spiritual, and they can be affected by the three *guṇas*: *sattva*, *rajas* and *tamas*.

5) *Smṛti*: Memory

This function helps us to be able to remember any form of experience. There are three types of memory: normal, abnormal and supernormal.

These five functions are inter-related. There is always some limitation operating in each function of mind. The process of concentration/meditation or mental integration requires thorough understanding of these functions.

The next page shows a Mind Wave Chart that explains mind waves and their positive and negative manifestations.

Mind Wave Chart

Mind Wave	Positive	Negative
Correct Perception Direct Indirect Inference	Unity • Oneness Love • Faith Compassion Understanding Living from Inner Truth Recognizing in others the positive values we see in ourselves	Forgetting our "Oneness" Self Deception Self Punishment Exaggerations of Fact Misleading Embellishment Perpetuating Stereotypes Withholding Truth
Incorrect Perception If we have an incorrect or distorted perception of ourselves, we project the same onto others and soon everything we perceive around us will begin to support incorrect perception. We can influence others based on our own distortions just as they may influence us from their own distorted or "incorrect" perceptions.		Twists and distorts facts Unjustly reactive Promotes misconceptions Suspicion Judgments based on misperception Territorialities Defensive Deceitful • Deceptive
Imagination Constructive Destructive	Visionary Creative New Ideas Inventive Translates spirit into reality	Projects images and expectations onto others Tries to live up to images and expectations OF others Need for acceptance Sacrifices integrity Conjures up conflicts that have no validity
Sleep Physical Psychological	Wakefulness Interest Enthusiasm for Life Being fully in the moment Waking up to who we really are	Boredom Tuning out Mental limitation on receptivity Going to sleep to our own possibilities
Memory Abnormal Normal Supernormal	Remembering our "oneness" with all of creation	Forgetfulness Senility • Amnesia Memory brings up everything that will support either our contracted or expansive consciousness

I.7 PRATYAKṢĀNUMĀNĀGAMĀḤ PRAMĀṆĀNI

***Pratyakṣa** = direct perception*
***Anumāna** = inference*
***Agamāḥ** = scriptural testimony*
***Pramāṇa** = source of right knowledge*
***Ani** = the three are*

Direct Experience, Indirect Experience And Inference Of Experience Of Others Constitute *Pramāṇa* Or Accurate And Correct Perception.

Pramāṇa: Correct Perception

Prā is to bring forth and *mana* means to think.
Pramāṇa is to bring forth the thinking mind.

The first non-painful mind wave is *pramāṇa* or correct, accurate or factual perception. There are three parts of *pramāṇa*: l) direct 2) indirect 3) inference of others.

1) Direct Experience

In direct experience, we perceive truth or right knowledge within relativity. An example would be that the stars look small to us from our world, but they are really huge. Although the stars are not really small, it is correct perception within relativity to experience the stars as small.

When we have a direct experience of that in which we had faith, it becomes a belief. Belief is the outgrowth of our own experience. Until then it is faith. Transformation of the intellect into intuitive knowledge is *śraddhā*, faith. We can have direct experience of the universal presence through a vision, an inner voice, a rapturous sensation or just a knowing or feeling of the universal presence of this eternal cosmic vibration.

2) Indirect Experience

The second aspect of *pramāṇa* is indirect experience. This includes taking the experience of another as our own. In indirect experience, we may believe there is a God because someone we know and trust has had a direct experience of the universal intelligence. Even though we have not had our own direct experience, if we resonate with this person's experience, we will believe in a higher power and take it on as if it were our own.

Someone may relate a bad experience they had with a person, and in hearing their story, we take on their experience as our own. However, if we were to meet that person, our own experience may be very different. If a friend has a negative experience with someone, it helps to "go direct." Your experience may be totally different than theirs.

3) Inference

Inference from others is like taking knowledge from the Bible, the Vedas and other religious books that have been passed down through the ages. Sometimes we can believe it as fact, but there can be mis-interpretation that we believe as fact. The further we get away from the source the more distortions that can happen. It is like the game of telephone. It is a long ways down the line from our own direct or indirect experience.

Examples of inference would be receiving information from news media, social media, internet, books and scriptures from the major world's religions. We may form our own beliefs based upon the direct experience of mystics, saints and sages who have been immortalized throughout the ages. We are usually drawn to those teachings that awaken within us a deep recognition of Truth, predicating our faith and beliefs on the inference of others. This third step of *pramāṇa*, (accurate perception) requires a high degree of discernment, discrimination and a highly developed sense of intuition.

If one does not share our perceptions correct or incorrect, we may criticize them for holding a different view. The essence of equanimity is to hold two or more perspectives simultaneously. Just as we move towards a balance of polarities in our physical bodies, we are aware of the balance in the mental and emotional bodies.

The further we get away from an accurate perception of our own direct experience, the more easily we can be conditioned by others. Most belief systems are formed and easily conditioned by cultural, societal and political systems of the times in which we live. It is difficult to sort out our individual perceptions from the collective belief systems that we have knowingly or unknowingly taken on as our own.

A government convinces their people that there is an enemy and we must declare war against them. The faces of "the enemy" are all painted with the same brush. Dehumanization of the enemy is one of the first steps of warfare. It helps mobilize the people of a country to support war against another. This is the inference of others.

However, in *pramāṇa*, if we could look into the face of the enemy in our own direct experience we would have an opportunity to perceive them as individuals rather than stereotypes. We would find that they have the same hopes, aspirations and dreams for a better life for their children and future generations, just as we do. We would hear the lighthearted sounds of their children playing that are just like ours. If we were to experience "the enemy" for ourselves, we may find the sound of laughter and tears is the same in any language. We would see the face of their children as our own; we would feel the tears of the mothers and grandmothers as our own tears; we would perceive fear and apprehension of fathers and sons whether it is the "enemy" or our own. We can only see another as ourselves if we go direct—and have our own experience to help undo the conditioning that we have been exposed to.

The further we stray from our own direct experience, the easier it is to be easily influenced by the views of others. Mob violence stems from inference of others. It can sweep us into supporting and doing things that transgress our own conscience and sense of what is right for us.

At the height of the cold war, I was invited to the Soviet Union. I thought it would be fun to go behind the Iron Curtain into what President Reagan called, "the evil empire." I didn't realize it, but I had succumbed to the conditioning in the U.S. in believing the Soviets *were* our enemy. The first day in the marketplace near Red Square in Moscow, a grandmother came up to me and asked if I was Italian. "No, American," I responded. Her shock was evident when she dropped to her knees on the cold ground, put up her hands in a prayer position and cried, "Americansky! Mir, Mir" meaning peace, peace. I lifted her up off the ground and without words bent way down to embrace her withered frame. As I placed my tearful cheek against hers, our tears mingled in the river of oneness. It was at that moment that we both transcended our fear and stereotypes of one another. Because I had the opportunity to look directly into the face of the enemy, I found only the friend.

This story illustrates the power of one's direct experience in helping us to overcome whatever images of separation we are holding towards anyone. Cold or hot wars are an extreme form of misperception based on conditioned reflexes of a culture. In accurate perception, when we look directly into the face of the "enemy" we will see only the face of a friend.

Even in direct perception, family members may have totally different perspectives of the same situation like the story of the blind men touching each part of the elephant thinking their part is the whole elephant.

EXERCISE:

Discuss or Journal on the Following Questions:

1) *In what areas of your life have your perceptions been influenced, either indirectly or through inference of others?*
2) *Have you formed a stereotype of an individual based on someone else's experiences? If so, please elaborate.*
3) *Have you had the opportunity "to go direct" and form your own impressions through your direct experience? When you have, has there been a difference in your own perceptions rather than your perceptions based on the experiences of others? Please give an example.*

NOTE: The further we are from our direct experience and rely on the experiences of others, the more it is possible that we can slip into the next mind wave, incorrect perception or viparyaya.

I.8 VIPARYAYO MITHYĀJÑĀNAM ATADRŪPA PRATIṢṬHAM

***Viparyaḥ** = misconception*
***Mithyā** = false, mistaken*
***Jñānam** = knowledge*
***Atad** = not on that*
***Rūpa** = form*
***Pratiṣṭham** = based*

Viparyaya, Or Illusion, Is False Knowledge Formed Out Of Something As Other Than What It Is.

VIPARYAYA: INCORRECT PERCEPTION

Vi means *to negate, par* means *to fill* and *yaya* is like *yeah, really do it!*

So in *viparyaya* we are *really* not filling, or *really* not seeing, *really* not perceiving. This is known as incorrect perception, or wrong knowledge that has a concrete basis

The classic example would be the illustration of the snake and the rope. We may alert our families our neighbors with our screams of a snake but when the light is turned on, all are relieved that it is not a snake, but only a rope. This is compared to how we may live our life with incorrect perceptions, where we mistake one thing for another. We may react with fear when we hear a noise in the house thinking it might be someone trying to break in. Upon closer examination, we may find it is only the wind blowing a branch of a bush or a tree, against the window.

Another common misconception is when we feel offended, ignored or discounted when a friend did not return our phone call, e-mail or text message. We may feel devalued thinking we are not important enough for their immediate reply. We may wonder, was it something I said that may have angered or hurt them?

Another example of *viparyaya* would be the classic story of the blind men all touching the different parts of the elephant. One, touching the leg and foot of the elephant says, "The elephant is like the trunk of a tree." The other touching the ear says, "No, the elephant is like a great fan." Another, touching the tail exclaims, "The elephant is like a soft brush!" Yet another feeling the tusk of the elephant says, "The elephant is smooth like ivory." Their misconceptions are based on something real, but they are taking their piece of the experience as the whole truth. We may live our life like this, thinking our part, our single personal experience, is the entire truth.

To help conquer this mind wave, we should see ourselves in everything and everything in ourselves. At that point we will become one with the universe and the "Lila," or the divine play of life.

Viparyaya, wrong perception, can build an incorrect story of a situation that is reinforced by the next mind wave, *vikalpa* or imagination.

EXERCISE:
Discuss or Journal:
1) *How has inference of others led you to perceive a situation incorrectly? Please give an example of viparyaya from your own life.*

I.9 ŚABDAJÑĀNĀNUPĀTĪ VASTU ŚŪNYO VIKALPAḤ

Śabda *= word, sound*
Jñāna *= knowledge*
Anupāti *= arises*
Vastu *= reality, real object*
Śūnyaḥ *= without any*
Vikalpaḥ *= verbal delusion*

The Modification Called *Vikalpa* Is Based On Verbal Cognition In Regards To Something That Does Not Exist.

VIKALPA: IMAGINATION

Vi is a Sanskrit prefix that reverses and negates the verb *kalpa,* which means *to be in the correct order or time sequence*. Therefore, *vikalpa* means *no time*.

This mind-wave is beyond time. It is the transcendence of time known as imagination. In our imagination, we can defy time projecting our mind anywhere beyond this moment. We can reach into the depths of the subconscious and pull up past memories and soar like a bird into the future. Neither the body, nor any other constraint in life limits the imagination. Through imagination we can manifest our greatest dreams. It builds edifices of art, music and technology. It inspires science and all bodies of knowledge as well as religious and spiritual guidelines.

Norman Vincent Peal said, "Imaging is a kind of laser beam of the imagination. It is a shaft of mental energy in which the desired goal or outcome is pictured so vividly by the conscious mind that the unconscious mind accepts it and is activated by it. This [the imagination] releases powerful internal forces that can bring about astonishing changes in the life of the person who is doing the imaging."

Swami Paramahamsa Yogānanda referred to imagination in his autobiography when he said, "God first created the earth as an idea. Then He quickened it; energy atoms came into being. He coordinated the atoms into this solid sphere. All its molecules are held together by the will of God. When this universal creative force withdraws its energy or will, the earth will disintegrate into pure energy. Energy will dissolve into consciousness and the earth-idea, will disappear from objectivity."

Imagination is a nation of images. There is a creative part to *vikalpa* but that aspect can be hidden and subdued by our confusion. When the *ahaṁkāra,* or ego distorts this wonderful mind wave, we project our images onto another and try to live up to the images that others have projected onto us. This of course breeds expectation. *Vikalpa* is the aspect of our mind that "falls" in love, not with another person, but with the image we are projecting onto that person. As long as they continue to live up to and enhance our images, we will love them. However, when they go on being who they are, we may become angry and tear them off the very pedestal that we ourselves placed them on. A yogi once said, "I don't care if you put me on a pedestal, just give me an elevator."

Imaging ... is a shaft of mental energy in which the desired goal or outcome is pictured so vividly by the conscious mind that the unconscious mind eventually accepts it and is activated by it. The imagination releases powerful internal forces that can bring about astonishing change in the life of the person who is doing the imaging

In *vikalpa* we also project our images onto a teacher or guru, a priest or minister or a politician. If any of their frailties or misconduct comes to light, bitterness, anger and even betrayal can result. In our disappointment, we are really blaming them for not living up to our expectations and the standards we have set for them. Imagination has caused the anger and bitterness, not the person themselves. We may seldom realize that expectations are a symptom and *vikalpa*, or imagination, is the cause.

According to the *Yoga Sūtras*, the essence of *yoga* is to, "still the fluctuations or waves that arise in the field of the *citta*." The following is a very common example of how *vikalpa* can create turbulence in the mind.

If our friend does not answer our calls and messages, we may use our imagination negatively to build on the foundation of incorrect perception to create elaborate stories of why they did not respond to our messages culminating in the essence of, "They don't love me." Feeling irrelevant, unseen and unloved, we may begin to build a case against them, finding all the reasons why we should be angry. The mind waves become more turbulent, thinking of all the reasons of why we should terminate the friendship and then escalating into angry projections of what they should say in retaliation. We rehearse the script, building the story into a crescendo of events. The storms of the mind engulf logic and reason until our friend calls, apologizing profusely that they were away and out of cell phone range and did not have access to email.

What a psycho-physiological storm we have passed through in that time! Our mind and in turn, its transmission of neuromuscular tension in the body, influences our physical health as well as our emotional wellbeing. The storms of our mind may have been raging for days, or weeks, wildly creating and rehearsing imaginary stories that had no validity in fact, or a shred of accurate perception, adding further to the distortion and creating pain for our selves. They had nothing to do with the great drama we created and enacted within our own mind. S.N. Goenka, the great *vipassanā* teacher said, "We keep playing out the drama that we stage within our own minds."

When our friend did not respond to us, we abused our self through the lens of *ahaṁkāra*, the ego. If our ego is *tamasic*, we pity our self, feeling unseen, unheard, irrelevant and not important enough to warrant a response. If our ego is *rajasic*, we go into anger, and place outward blame onto the friend, finding the faults in the friend. The *sattvic* ego might look at it differently. The *sattvic* ego has transcended its own individuation to see a greater perspective like the *buddhi* mind. It goes on with its life, putting the incidence on the back burner and holds the space for the friend to respond when they can. It does not blame or condemn, feel self-pity or unworthiness. It knows that it is part of a greater consciousness and holds all in the substratum of its being.

The *buddhi* is benevolent and compassionate. It does not need to forgive anyone because it never blamed. It does not trespass into the space of another because it does not superimpose its own agenda even when they are superimposing their outer projections onto us. It has no expectation of what another must do and say, and as a result does not become attached to an outcome. This is *sattvic* ego, the *buddhi* mind, where we transform the more contracted parts of the ego into a more expanded aspect of over-mind that sees all sides of a situation. It is at peace in itself and in turn with the world around. The mind finds greater clarity and stillness. We don't have to retreat to a mountaintop but can find it in the marketplace of life.

Whenever I think of *vikalpa*, I think of a part of the Lord's Prayer. "Forgive us our trespasses as we forgive others for trespassing against us." If the *ahaṁkāra*, or ego part of mind, crosses the border and invades the space of another through judgment, criticism or condemnation, it is a form of trespassing. We are invading the territory of another without being invited. Just as we may do this individually, we can also do this collectively as nations.

A vision without a task is but a dream.
A task without a vision is drudgery.
A vision with a task can change the world

Vikalpa can even be applied to the subject of terrorism in the world. Instead of seeing the terrorists outside of ourselves, can we see the terrorist within our self? This expresses itself in combativeness and the desire to create dissention and/or the desire to destroy our own creations. This can happen at the level of business when someone builds an organization and when no longer useful in that organization there is a desire to destroy the very thing that they created. This is the self-important ego's desire to control in order to support its own identity. This causes them to contract rather than expand and leads to more separation rather than unification.

In *vikalpa*, we may protect self-image. This reflects in our resistance to associate with "certain people" for fear of tarnishing our own image personally and/or politically. There are times when we may be afraid to speak out for what we believe for fear we won't be approved of. "What will others think?" Others influence our thinking more than we realize. *Vikalpa* or imagination can be seen in the form of peer pressure. We conform to the beliefs of others so that we will be accepted and not excluded by our associates.

The mind wave of *vikalpa* when tainted by the ego, tries to please others and to seek their approval, even if it means straying from our own inner core beliefs and what is true to our inner being. When this happens, we begin to do what we *think* we should be doing instead of doing what we *know* we should be doing. As we stray from our own center of balance in trying to live up to the images projected onto us, we may grow increasingly resentful and angry of the very person or persons we are trying to please — including ourselves.

Vikalpa is not only that part of our mind wave that projects its images onto another, it also tries to live up to the images others may have knowingly or unknowingly projected onto us. We may feel like a failure if we don't live up to the expectations of others. We see this in children who, in seeking approval, may try to live up to the spoken or unspoken expectation of the parents.

Why do we get nervous when we have to speak in front of a group of people? It seems as if nervousness could be part of *vikalpa* when we try to live up to the expectations and the images that others are projecting onto us. We may knowingly or unknowingly desire to have audience approval. "How will they respond to what I am presenting? What if they don't like me? What if? What if?" If the ego mind is in the driver's seat of the chariot, through the imagination of *vikalpa*, it usually perceives separation and hungers for approval. It wants to present a likeable image and seeks approval of its own separative self. It wants to be assured and reassured that it is loved.

If we were in the *buddhi* mind, we would be unattached to the outcome. There would be no anxiety or nervousness in teaching or presenting in front of people. We would do our best in the presentation and then let go of any desired outcome. We would not be affected by thoughts of, "Did they like me? Or was it awful?" We would be unaffected by other people's opinions, good, bad, indifferent or neutral. Ultimately, we seek approval because we subconsciously want to know that we are loved and seen and at one with our audience.

In *vikalpa* we may take an action, not for the sake of the action but because we want something from it. We may uphold an image of ourselves wanting recognition, respect, approval, love, and appreciation from others. This would be a questionable and impure motive for our actions in life.

> *"God first created the earth as an idea ... all its molecules are held together by the will of God.*
>
> *When this universal creative force withdraws its energy or will, the earth will disintegrate into pure energy.*
>
> *Energy will dissolve into consciousness and the earth-idea, will disappear from objectivity."*
>
> *- Paramahamsa Yogananda*

Years ago, a *Yoga Sūtra* student was asked to observe how *vikalpa* would manifest in the coming week in her life. At the end of the week, she came back to class with a clear example of *vikalpa*. She hadn't seen her friends for nine years and they were coming to see her. She wanted them to see how good she looked since they last saw her and wanted to revel in their compliments. She went to the beauty shop, learned how to apply makeup, and bought new clothes to present the very best image of herself that she could. Just before they arrived, her horse escaped from the barn. As she put it back in its stall, she slipped in the mud that was now splattered all over her new clothes. She was angry at the horse because it destroyed the image she wanted to portray to her friends. She wasn't concentrating on the moment and in trying to put the horse into its stall, it kicked her in the face. Her face quickly became bruised and swollen. She said that it took the kick in the face to "wake her up" and finally let go of the image her ego was trying to create.

She was actually able to observe *vikalpa* as one image after another was destroyed. When the horse kicked her in the face, she felt it was the hand of God reminding her to come back to center, and let go of trying to build and protect her self-image. She laughed saying she would never forget to observe the images she tried to uphold of herself in the eyes of others and would become more vigilant of not projecting images onto others. When she relayed this story, I thought of William Shakespeare who wrote "there is a point where tragedy becomes so tragic it becomes comedy."

Part of the practice of *yoga* in *āsana* and life's poses is staying centered in the midst of the polarities of opposites such as praise or blame, success or failure, criticism or compliment. In the *Yoga Sūtras*, there is a reoccurring theme of self-responsibility, not self-blame. "We are all the arcitects of our own destiny."

We Are All Architects of Our Own Destiny

Vikalpa is a major mind wave that is difficult to tame. Awareness and self-observation help to hold our center in the midst of life's storms and the nation of images that surround us. If we can hold our mind and thoughts in a state of equanimity, we won't criticize others for having a differing view or perspective. The essence of equanimity is holding two or more perspectives simultaneously. Just as we move towards a balance of polarities in our physical body, it also brings balance to the mental and emotional bodies. By holding all others in the light of "oneness," we will see their journey as our own.

EXERCISE:

Please Discuss or Journal on the Following Questions:

1) *Write about how vikalpa manifests in your life.*
2) *Please list both positive and negative images you are projecting onto a:*
    a) *politician*
    b) *celebrity*
    c) *friend*
    d) *family member/s*
    e) *challenging relationship*
    f) *yourself*
3) *What images have been imposed on you that you have tried to live up to?*
4) *Discuss the main issues in your life that create disturbances and oscillation in the waves of your mind.*

HOMEPLAY: *For one week observe vikalpa as you go about daily activities. Write your observations in your sūtra diary each night.*

I.10 ABHĀVA PRATYAYĀLAMBANĀ VṚTTIR NIDRĀ

Abhāva = *nothingness*
Pratyaya = *cognition*
Alambanā = *support*
Vṛttiḥ = *modification of the mind*
Nidrā = *sleep*

That Mental Modificiation Supported By Cognition Of Nothingness Is Sleep.

NIDRĀ (SLEEP)

Sleep is a gateway to the subconscious and unconscious depths of the mind. When we close the outer eyes, the inner eye opens. Wherever we place our attention, energy follows. In the waking state, it is said that consciousness is centered between the brows in the *ajña cakra*. In sleeping, consciousness moves toward the heart center, the *anāhata cakra*. In dreaming, our consciousness moves to the throat center, the *viśuddhi cakra*. The throat center detaches the ego from the body. In the sleep state, the senses are withdrawn from the mind and the mind is withdrawn into the heart. This withdrawal is brought about by the functions of *puritat nāḍī* in the heart center. The *puritat* is related to the pericardium, which is the covering that surrounds the lotus of the heart. The *nāḍīs* are subtle astral channels that correspond to the physical nervous system.

Sleep reveals the bliss of the Self. There are three forms of sleep:
l) physical 2) psychological and 3) spiritual.

PHYSICAL SLEEP is a necessity for physical health and vitality. When the *citta* (the mind stuff) withdraws itself from the central nervous system, the head drops and the spine can no longer remain erect and thus, physical sleep is usually in a reclining position. Physical sleep is nature's tonic that cleanses the brain tissue, relaxes the nervous system and refreshes the mind. It brings about recuperative and healing effects of both body and mind.

On a subtle level, there is a gateway in the brain between the frontal and posterior lobes. When our eyes are open and we project our senses during the day, the *prāṇic* energy is propelled forward. At night when it grows dark and our eyes are closed, the energy automatically swings to the sleep center in the back of the brain. Towards dawn the energy begins to shift to the frontal lobes, opening the eyes and activating the conscious mind to prepare for the day's activities with the light of dawn as a stimulant for the sensory organs or the conscious mind. Night is the time when the conscious mind (the rational mind that makes order out of things) shuts down. *Citta*, or subconscious, then becomes more active, giving rise to the *vikalpa*, imagination, where the mind can create anything beyond time, space or rationality. Dreams are not created; they reveal the storehouse of impressions deep within the layers of the *citta* or psyche. Dreams are revelations of the present and reflect past experiences, even past life experience. Dreams can also project into the future as they transcend boundaries of time and space.

Swami Jyotirmayānanda says, "The art of sound sleep is important in the life of a *yogin*. There is a difference between unhealthy sleep and a profound movement of sleep as part of the soul's evolution. An unhealthy sleep produced by drugs is detrimental for one's physical and mental health. The ability to control one's sleep according to one's will is considered a great Yogic achievement. It is an expression of a very high level of personality integration." In healthy sleep, it is possible to control sleep patterns without depriving oneself from sleeping. Rather the yogi uses sleep as a mystical entrance into the deeper layers of the subconscious. The art of sleep becomes a means to an end.

Swami Jyotirmayānanda has said from a Vedantic perspective that, "Sleep reveals the bliss of the Self through a dark veil of ignorance. A person is free from the duality of the world and free from the experiences of multiplicity, free from all relations and relatives from debt and worry. Yet, in sleep one can be deeply immersed in their own bliss. Therefore, sleep reveals the fact of the blissful nature of the Self."

Swamiji has taught, "Sleep is considered to be a rehearsal for death. Death reveals the fact of the cessation of the world phenomena. It is the psychological confrontation of death which creates a sense of pathos, terror and agony; but the actual movement in death is joyous, desirable, and relaxing." In a healthy sleep, nature can rehearse a variety of perspectives of self-realization.

Vedāntic philosophers group sleep (*suṣupti*) and death in one category, "Death is a greater process of sleep. During death, the senses are withdrawn into the mind. Even the *prāṇas* or the vital forces are withdrawn into the mind. This is the difference between sleep and death. During sleep, the *prāṇas* continue to guard the body until the mind returns to it. But during death the mind moves towards the heart along with the *prāṇas* and the senses."

A comatose state is considered to be midway point between sleep and death. The *prāṇas* are partially withdrawn during the coma but due to the presence of life-sustaining *karma*, they return again in the same body. The soul might see the portals of death but comes back to its day-to-day life.

In Buddhism as well, it has been said that sleep is the rehearsal for death. The way we train our thread of consciousness to remain aware even while we sleep is a rehearsal for holding the consciousness steady as one travels through a myriad of experiences in their journey when the soul leaves the body. Again in that state it is learning to remain centered between the waking and sleeping state. I call this sleep in looking through the closed eyelids. It is a state where even though the eyes are closed, you can see everything in the room and even throughout every room of the house and even the building and grounds outside the house. I have found that theta wave or hypnagogic imagery state is like moving from the confines of third dimensional consciousness into a more expanded realm of the fourth, and sometimes fifth dimensional consciousness. It is a form of time travel; in this state, we transform intellect into intuition.

In this state, brilliant ideas form and before dropping into the luxury of a deep sleep we say to ourselves that we must remember this in the morning. However, upon awakening it's many times forgotten, like the journey through the birth canal when we forget what was on the other side.

Insomnia is becoming an epidemic in our culture. So much of the activities of modern society over-stimulate the sympathetic nervous system, which stimulates frontal brain activity. Television, computers, cell phones, and smart phones are all just some of the reasons for our frontal brain stimulation. Lack of exercise and caffeine in our foods and drinks all act to stimulate the frontal lobes of the brain making it difficult for *prāṇa* to swing back to the posterior lobes at night. Lack of sleep for long periods of time can cause, on a very subtle level, the gateway between frontal and posterior or conscious and subconscious mind to close, giving a sensation as if the *prāṇa*, or energy, is trapped in the frontal lobes. It takes a great deal of discipline and awareness to retrain the brain to once more come into balance. It can be done with *āsana* practice designed to stimulate the posterior nerves of the spine, which stimulates the parasympathetic nervous.

Helpful Tips for Insomnia:

- *Forward Bends, Bridge Pose and Half Plow with legs over a chair are helpful to stimulate the parasympathetic nervous system before bed.*
- *Avoid backbends and other inverted poses in the evening.*
- *Taking magnesium helps to relax the body at night.*
- *Relaxation techniques and yoga nidrā can be very helpful.*

BRAINWAVE STATES AND DREAMS

The fourth mind wave, sleep or *nidrā* has multiple layers. There are varying levels of sleep based on the waves of mind:

1) Beta wave – wakefulness
2) Alpha wave – relaxed and calm state of mind
3) Theta wave – state of mind between the waking and sleeping. It is the hypnagogic state where brilliant ideas come to the surface of the mind. It is a state of meditation where mind is balanced between the conscious and subconscious. This is the state that Albert Einstein was said to live in.
4) Delta waves – deep sleep, unconscious where dreams can surface. When the conscious mind is "asleep" dreams may arise. Dreams come from *vikalpa* or imagination. When the conscious mind is out of the way, distortions of past experiences may manifest. These dreams can be due to past experiences stored in the psyche and/or images that may manifest in future wakeful states. Dreams can help us work out various life's challenges as well as give premonitions of things to come.

These can relate to the Vedic view of the brainwave states:

1) *jāgrat* – all conscious actions in a wakeful state
2) *svapnā* – all actions in the sleep stage; non wakeful
3) *suṣupti* – all actions in the trance state, deep sleep, deeply meditative

NOTE: Scientists have discovered gamma waves, which vibrate at such a high frequency, it's possible they can become still. This takes the mind into that state of 'citta vṛtti nirodaḥ.'

Meditation and *yoga* can bring us into the state where the *manas* mind of sensory perceptions is functioning in equal balance as the subconscious layers of the *citta*. When they are in unison whether in a meditative seat, in *āsana* practice, with our breath, chanting, etc. we can enter into the theta wave state. There is a mystic marriage of the frontal and posterior lobes of our brain in between the pituitary, which is connected to the optic nerve and activates conscious mind and the pineal, towards the back of the brain which relates to the subconscious mind. These spatial receptors in our brain represent respectively the masculine and feminine, the *ha* and *ṭha*, the sun and moon. The essence of *yoga* is to bring about an androgynous balance of these two polarities that not only exist within nature, but also in our own bodies. At night as the energy shifts from the front to the back brain, we can train ourselves to linger in the space between these two opposites, before the delta waves become prominent.

Swami Paramahamsa Yogānanda mentions in his autobiography that the substance of a dream is held in materialization by the subconscious thoughts of the dreamer. When that cohesive thought is withdrawn in wakefulness, the dreamer and its elements dissolve. When we close our eyes we erect a dream creation, which on awakening effortlessly dematerializes. This follows the Divine archetypical pattern; when we awaken to the Cosmic Consciousness, the illusion of separation dematerializes. In the *yoga* philosophy, it is believed that the earth and the entire cosmos were created out of an idea. This reminds me of the children's song that ends with, "Life is but a dream." Are we the dream or the dreamer? Are we the creation or the creator? It is said that what is night to the ordinary man is day to the *yogi* and what is day to the worldly person is night to a *yogin*.

EXERCISE:

Please Discuss or Journal on the Following Questions:

1) *What are your physical sleep patterns?*
2) *What are your dream patterns?*
3) *What does it mean that night to the ordinary man is day to the yogi? What is day to the worldly person and night to a yogin?*

PSYCHOLOGICAL SLEEP precedes physical sleep. Physical and psychological are interconnected. When the mind says enough is enough, it begins to withdraw itself from the central nervous system. The eyelids begin to droop, the *prāṇa* of the eyes withdraw from the external world and the ears no longer discern the sounds that are around. Since the conscious or rational mind is withdrawn, sound and images emerge out of the subconscious mind.

Psychological sleep is a means of avoidance. It is looking at something and not seeing. It is a dullness of mind, or a tuning out due to lack of concentration. We tune out to that which we don't want to see or hear. A part of our consciousness may also be conditioned to believe it's had enough and it loses its alertness to the moment. When we feel on "overload" and the mind thinks it has taken in enough, it shuts itself down figuratively or literally.

In psychological sleep, we are not "Being here now," as Ram Das would say. Our body may be present in a meeting but the mind may lose its focus, grow bored and use its imagination (*vikalpa*) to soar to great heights and time travel through flights of fancy and fantasy. The mind is obviously not in the moment. This can create a schism between mind and body. Or the mind can grow so dull that it internalizes itself lingering on the razor's edge of physical sleep. Anything that clouds the mind is considered to be a form of psychological sleep that can lead to a variety of forms of insulating or numbing oneself. Some "tune out" through alcohol and drugs (legal or illegal). It's interesting to note that the very substances we may take to enhance consciousness begin to cloud the mind rather than clear it. Food addictions may also be a contributing factor to psychological sleep. Spending hours in front of the television, computer or smart phones is another form of tuning out or going into psychological sleep. It's interesting to note that the very things we use to numb our feelings and end our pain become the very things that can create more pain.

Psychological sleep is reminiscent of the *sūtra* commentary, "The world is painful to the wise." When we awaken, and come out of psychological sleep, we may feel our own and others' pain. This pain can either inspire us to serve in order to alleviate the suffering of humanity or may cause us to seek variety of ways to avoid, withdraw, and not face into a situation as a way of "dealing" with pain.

Psychological sleep is becoming a situation that may need our attention. It can be denial or not addressing deeper issues within our selves and with others. We shut down our sensory intake, "I don't want to hear anymore," or "I don't want to see, I don't want to know." This can have a physiological affect upon the sensory organs. Eye muscles and tendons can be affected where the eyes can no longer see clearly either up close or far away. And the inner ear begins to harden over the years, shutting out the deeper subtleties of sounds and the voices of others. It's possible that this could even lead to memory disorders, which relate to the next section on memory.

Psychological sleep numbs itself and seeks addictions that help lessen the intensity of "feeling." It pulls away and veils itself from correct or accurate perception. We all want to find a way out of pain. Some choose *bhoga* (sense enjoyment) and others choose *yoga*.

EXERCISE:

Please Discuss or Journal on the Following Questions:

1) *What areas of your life are you ignoring and avoiding?*
2) *Who have you been avoiding and why?*
3) *Are you overdoing in one area of life and subconsciously avoiding another? If yes, please explain.*
4) *How is this revealed in your āsana practice?*
5) *Where are you overdoing and where are you under-doing?*

SPIRITUAL SLEEP is related to *avidyā*, ignorance, which is not seeing the nature of our oneness with our creator. This universal form of sleep is the basis of the "long dream" of the world-process. Ignorance or *avidyā* becomes the basis for experiencing numerous cycles of birth and death. In spiritual sleep when a yogi develops intuitive knowledge in *samādhi*, he or she dissolves the veil of ignorance and wakes up in recognition of its essential nature and realizes, "I am Brahman, the absolute." Until this realization dawns in one's consciousness, a soul is constantly sleeping in the night of ignorance. To awaken from this sleep is the essence of all *yoga*.

There is a thin line between sleep and samādhi

There is a thin line between sleep and *samādhi*. If our body holds a pose and consciousness drifts and slips into a state where we are halfway between the waking and sleeping state, it is usually *samādhi*. If we hold a pose and our consciousness drifts and the body sags or falls out of the pose, it is usually sleep. *Āsanas* and *mudrās* determine whether we are in sleep or *samādhi*. In *samādhi*, there arises an experience of the inner glory of the transcendental Self. The ego is transformed and wisdom shines forth. In sleep, the state of the ego remains unaltered.

Baba Haridas, the silent sage many years ago, wrote that, "In the awakened state, *rajas guṇa* predominates and the *vṛttis* or mind waves turn outward toward the world process. In the dream state, *rajas guṇa* is also present but it's covered by *tamas guṇa*, which turns the *vṛttis* inward. When *rajas guṇa* is present it creates dreams. The *tamas guṇa* in the dream state creates sleep first of all and then it keeps the mind, the thoughts from going out. It is the *tamas guṇa* that keeps the *vṛttis* turning inward, by sheer force of inertia, and gravity holds them there.

"In the dreamless state, *tamas guṇa* predominates and completely suppresses and overpowers the *rajas guṇa*. So there remains a thought-wave, a *vṛtti* of nothingness. Just as the thought waves turn inward due to *tamas guṇa*; in the same way, the *vṛttis* can be consciously turned inward by meditation by using *sattva guṇa* in place of *tamas guṇa*. In *sattva guṇa*, one-pointedness of mind can develop so deep that all *vṛttis* will be stopped. Pure *sattva* is actionless just like pure *tamas* is actionless. It's the quality of our consciousness that separates the two."

Swami Jyotirmayānada says, "The ability to control one's sleep according to one's will is considered a great *yogic* achievement."

In meditation one can reenact the deep sleep by balancing the *rajas* and *tamas* to come into a *sattvic* state of awareness. In dreamless sleep, all *vṛttis* are stopped by predominantly the *tamas guṇa*. Dreams transport us into another dimension that transcends the barriers of time. Sometimes we move in reverse to experience what was—in this life or another. In dreams, when the conscious mind is out of the way, we can fast forward to dimensions where we can even view future events. We might call it astral travel, where one can slip into the 4th dimension and come back and actually predict the future.

> *"The Ability to Control One's Sleep According to One's Will is Considered a Great Yogic Acheivement"*
>
> *-Swami Jyotirmayānanda*

Swami Jyotirmayānanda speaks at length about mystic sleep: "Sages who have destroyed the possibility of future embodiment are ever immersed in the ocean of bliss. Drunk as it were with the intoxicating nectar of immortality, they are no longer concerned with actions that have been performed or with actions that have not been performed. They move through the world with a childlike simplicity. Although they seem to accept the objects of the world, they are actually totally detached from them. In the state of mystic sleep, they are neither involved in avoiding conditions of adversity nor with promoting conditions of prosperity. They do not rejoice at the success of their activities nor do they grieve at their failures. The sun may turn cool and the moon may emit scorching heat and the flames of fire may burn downward, but the mind of the sage is not agitated by any sense of wonder. The mystic sleep is having realized the Self who is the wonder of wonders.

"In that state one is not affected by the happenings of the illusory world. Just as different dream creations appear and disappear at short intervals in the mind of a person who is sleeping at night, in the same manner, various conditions and circumstances appear and disappear during the sleep of ignorance. For the sage who is awake, all these become illusory."

Some individuals in their sleep transcend third dimensional confines of consciousness to experience personal or global events in their dreams that can be prophetic of the future.

Yoga nidrā is the yogic sleep where the body is asleep but the mind is awake. It is that place where the *prāṇa* in the pituitary gland is drawn back toward the cradle of the back of the skull to meet with the energies of the pineal. This is considered to be a mystic marriage of the masculine of the front brain and the feminine of the back brain. When these two are balanced, we move into the hypnagogic imagery state — a catalyst to awaken *ājñā* as well as *sahasrāra cakras*. This divine meeting of the *prāṇas* of the pituitary and pineal leads to the mystical sleep of *yoga nidrā. Yoga nidrā* is a very deep sleep, where one remains in theta wave state between waking, dreaming and sleeping state. Originally this was taught where the teacher makes sure the students do not drop into the delta state, where the mind sleeps. Instead they made sure the student was in that stage where the mind is awake as the body sleeps.

Yoga nidrā was originally taught as a form of "initiation" where the student was taken into the different levels of the *cakras* where each represents a different *loka* or plane of consciousness. Depending upon the *karma* of the student one can either enter into a more contractive or expansive consciousness. The practice of *yoga nidrā* can unveil future and past lives and reveal what has brought us to this present life. It is a very deep state of entering into other realms of consciousness and must have a highly qualified teacher to make sure that one can re-enter back into the body in this third dimension. Perhaps this is why, the essence and depth of *yoga nidrā* are not taught today in our society.

HOMEPLAY:

1) *Keep a journal of sleep patterns, night dreams and daydreams.*
2) *Observe in what areas of life you psychologically tune out.*
3) *In your meditations and āsanas can you observe that place between sleep and samādhi?*

I.11 ANUBHŪTA VIṢAYĀSAṂPRAMOṢAḤ SMṚTIḤ

Anu *= to flow along with*
Bhūta *= elements*
Viṣaya *= objects*
Asaṃpramoṣaḥ *= not forgotten*
Smṛtiḥ *= memory*

When A Mental Modification Of An Object Previously Experienced And Not Forgotten Comes Back To Consciousness — That is Memory.

I would translate this as:

Memory Is Not Allowing An Object That Has Been Experienced To Escape.

SMṚTI: MEMORY

The root verb of *smṛti* is *sma,* which means *to remember* or *to recall* and *ṛ* means *to rise upwards* from the unseen depths of the storehouse of the mind, which is the *citta*, the subconscious part of mind.

Swami Jyotirmayānanda says, "Memory is the function of the mind that revives the experience of the past. This enables one to seek the cause of limitation, the roots of our weaknesses, and aids in the integration of the personality."

Memory is a bank or reservoir of impressions created by previous actions or experiences. It is an accumulation and registry of these series of events we call "life." It is the registry and depository of the *citta* and its many layers, from the preconscious to the subconscious and collective unconscious.

Memories bury themselves in the chambers of the psyche. The deeper the impression of an experience, the deeper is the impression in the vaults of memory. In *smṛti*, we are bringing up the member or part once again and this is called to "re-member." As the *sūtra* says, "Memory is not allowing an object or experience to escape." Every conscious experience becomes a subconscious impression and as Mr. B.K.S. Iyengar has said, "The invisible must become visible before it can be eradicated," or as I prefer to say, transformed.

> *"A possessor of a memory gets to travel in time and in telling their stories, they incant it back into existence."*
>
> *Swami Jyotirmayānanda*

Dr. Karl Pribram, Stanford surgeon and neuroscientist, has described the brain as a holographic storage network in which memory is imprinted in waveforms and distributed throughout the entire brain, not simply stored in just one area. Dr. Pribram believes that a stimulus of sound, color or taste, can trigger brain mechanisms that instantly sift through and shape the appropriate waves into a rich three-dimensional memory.

When we vividly imagine running, there are small but measurable contractions in our muscles, comparable to the changes that occur during actual running. When visualizing an *āsana* before taking the pose, students have said that the pose came more easily when in the pose. According to Doctor Pribam, "what you're doing with this visualization is flooding the brain and nervous system with a pure, specific sensory vision of what we desire. When we do that, our research shows that the electrochemistry of the brain incorporates this vision in all its detail as if we had already accomplished our goal. It becomes so real that it's imprinted that way within the brain." For decades in *yoga* we would simply say, when thought takes form, it becomes an action.

Most experiences in life will register as an impression in the subconscious. These are known as *saṃskāras* and are intimately connected with memory. These impressions may be as light as the touch of a feather floating upon the surface of the waters of the mind, never penetrating its depths, never creating a wave or a ripple. These impressions can easily be recalled from the layer of the preconscious mind. Other memories are like a straw that floats for a time on the surface until it absorbs the water and slowly floats downward but doesn't drop all the way to the bottom. Other impressions are like a pebble, and others like a boulder that finds its way to the deeper layers of the psyche.

Some impressions are chiseled in granite leaving indelible grooves. These deeper impressions that take a longer time to manifest are known as *vāsanās*. *Vāsanās* are stored in the deepest part of the subconscious memory. They are like the undertow of the ocean. These impressions may, as the *yoga* teachings say, take a few lifetimes to manifest. They are more difficult to "see" in the milky ocean of the mind. Perhaps this is why Sri Aurobindo Gosh referred to *yoga* as "compressed evolution." We don't wait for the accumulated memories to reveal themselves but we take the practices that open the channels and clarify the hidden parts of mind so they can bubble up to the surface of the conscious mind more quickly. "The invisible must become visible before it can be eradicated." When these memories emerge, whether pleasurable or un-pleasurable, they can create a sense of cellular lightness where the weight of past memories are lifted and no longer hold us back from whom and what we truly are.

Memories of things that are real are *pramāṇa*—correct perception. Memories of things that are unreal are *viparyaya*—incorrect perception.

Memory can be sometimes dull and sometimes healthy. When healthy it lifts us above the limitations of life. When it is bright it awakens experiences in life that lead to evolutionary enfoldment of one's remembrance. If dull it keeps the mind involved in the revival of discordant and fragmentary experiences leading to confusion. When healthy we transcend life's limitations but when diseased one cannot have accurate perception. Fact and fiction get turned around with the help of the embellishments of the imaginations or daydreams. The facts become distorted and through psychological sleep we negate the accuracy of events and create mental complexes and miseries each time we repeat a thought. The mental modifications become turbulent and the mind cannot come to rest. Many people use memory to cling to the memories of the past and grasp for the expectations of the future.

Many people use memory to cling to the memories of the past and grasp for the expectations of the future

The memory of the transcendent Self is buried in all of us. This memory brings us to these teachings; it brings us to an awakened soul who reminds us of what we already know. Like *amṛta*, the nectar of our own immortality that lies buried in the human heart, it awakens, taking us out of the sleep of our mortal self, into the remembrance of what we have never forgotten. We are not this mind or passing personality but we are one with the immortal source.

As one becomes chronologically older in earth's timetables, it becomes easier to look back than to look ahead. We have vast storehouses of past experiences. If we linger and rehash the negative experiences, it produces a contractive consciousness and in turn pain. If we look at the wonderful and exciting memories of the past, it too can be painful because those high points of life are not currently happening. It can also be painful to remember our loved ones who may no longer be in this dimension in the form we were accustomed to. Even the most precious memories contain the seeds of pain. In memory, we compare the past to the present or a future moment. There is a hidden part of human nature that wants to keep the status quo and fend off change because it can bring pain.

Dr. Haridas Chaudhuri, founder of the California Institute for Integral Studies, would ask his students if it was possible to bathe in the same waters of the Ganges twice. After swimming in the swift waters near the source of the Ganges, it seemed almost impossible to bathe in the same waters even once.

"Anicha, anicha," as the Buddhist say, "changing, changing." Yet memory can crystallize an event or a person, by locking them into an unchanging form whether it is positive or negative.

Due to the imagination of *vikalpa*, when an event occurs, the imagination can embellish it and it deposits itself in the banks of memory as a positive or negative experience. If we have a negative experience of an individual, we might always throughout our lifetime, crystallize a contractive thought or negative image of that person. We may not allow a change of mind and heart, even though that person is continually changing. This begins to influence our own mind and even our body. Some *yogis* believe that crystallization in our memory can create growing stiffness in our body. In *yoga* and *Āyurveda* it is said that body *is* crystallized mind.

It is in memory that we find the roots of fear (II:9). The *Yoga Sūtras* intimate, "We cannot fear anything we have not previously experienced." We can see here how this fifth *vṛtti* of memory correlates to the fifth *kleśa* of fear. Due to memory of past negative experiences in a relationship, one would be reluctant and even fearful to enter into another relationship. They may be afraid that it could cause a repetition of emotional pain previously experienced.

What makes the mind wave of *smṛti* or memory become painful? The *ahaṁkāra* of ego loves to create havoc and stir up the storms of the mind. The details of even this present life can be distorted or not remembered at all. However, the mind stores all records of all experiences in this mysterious vault of *smṛti*.

There are 3 forms of memory l) abnormal, 2) normal, 3) supernormal.

ABNORMAL MEMORY

If we have been ignoring something, not wanting to look at it as in psychological sleep, it can become more deeply embedded in the deeper layers of mind with the passing of time. This repression of the impression will drop to the deeper and deepest layers of the psyche in the *citta* and create an undertow of chronic turbulence that impacts our bodies as well as mind. When we are burdened in the *citta*, we find we can't remember.

The more we tune out in psychological sleep, the more we shut down. Psychological sleep eventually impairs the memory. It is a form of repression, shutting out what we do not want to see or hear. This can eventually impair our sensory organs such as eyes or ears, impede circulative fluids and harden tissues. A person who is hard of hearing will at times have 'selective hearing,' when they hear only what they choose to hear. When we continue to repress in psychological sleep, it will eventually have an impact upon our memory. When we are fully awake and interested in something, we will remember. It's like having a treasure map to the place where gold is buried; we're excited and want to remember the site.

When we tune out or slip into psychological sleep we are like sleepwalkers or somnambulists moving through life in the fog of the dream we have woven for ourselves. This eventually impairs our memory, escalating forgetfulness, which has many layers, from 'senior moments' to forgetting the associations of those closest to us in life and finally the forgetfulness of oneself. In *yoga,* the idea is to be in the moment. Those with Alzeimer's disease are in the moment, but this is not the desired state of *yoga*. In *yoga*, being in the moment means being in focused clarity. Frustration, agitation, helplessness and fear are not the desired states of clarity. In the desired yogic state of clarity, they can care for themselves and contribute to a sense of peace, empowerment and connection to the world and to the Divine source.

Many times when a person undergoes a deep trauma like sexual abuse, it is wiped clean from the conscious memory because the mind is not ready to face it. As a form of psychological sleep, the memory is pushed into the deeper recesses of the subconscious mind (*citta*). Years later, when one feels safe, a *yoga* practice or body therapy can unleash the memory into the conscious mind and the person will remember something they never before realized had happened in their life. The memory was held all that time in the subconscious until brought to the surface for healing and release.

We do not remember many of our experiences, even in the present life. Some we do not want to remember and some we do. No matter how much we want to throw some memories out, we cannot discard them. Abnormal memory distorts past experience due to imagination, misconception and psychological sleep (inertia). The results are a burdened subconscious, memory disorders, faulty reason and ego. This causes a state of the mind in which there is dullness of mental functions and one is internally worried and preoccupied. This can cause a variety of degrees of memory loss that yogis consider a form of subconscious obstructions.

Reasons for lapse of memory:

1) inaccurate perception or misconceptions resulting in a dull mind,
2) gap of a considerable time period,
3) change of condition or environment,
4) confused ideation, and
5) absence of enthusiasm or excitement.

One thing that will improve our memory is being on fire with finding our life's work!

Abnormal memory also reflects a dullness of the mental functions, internal preoccupation that again, is a form of psychological sleep. Abnormal memory is also linked to the *vṛtti* of *viparyaya* or misconception. It has a distorted view of reality and can act as an obstacle to one's own human potential.

NORMAL MEMORY

Normal memory does not exaggerate or distort life's circumstances. It can face the realities of life with poise and clarity. It remembers and uses past events to act as a springboard for the future. This form of memory has fewer dreams and aids us in *yoga* practice. Normal memory would include a "good memory." Usually we have a good memory if we try not to exaggerate and distort facts. Good memory comes from an alert and interested mind. If it is interested in a topic it will not wander and get caught in the labyrinth of a circuitous and scattered mind. It may periodically "check out" at times, lapsing into psychological sleep but it is brief and temporary. Normal memory builds upon its healthy foundations of the past.

> *"Memory is the function of the mind that revives the experience of the past. This enables one to seek the cause of limitation, the roots of our weaknesses and aids in the integration of the personality."*
>
> *Swami Jyotirmayāndanda*

The power of memory and its contents of experiences arise from the storehouse of impressions, the *citta*. One's own inner evolution will determine if remembrances extend beyond the womb. Memories of past lives may emerge or not. For one's spiritual unfolding, it is not important or necessary to remember and try to dredge up memories of previous personalities. We have enough accumulation of memories in this life. It is not important for the soul to carry the burden of the previous impressions. The soul, which regulates the power of memory and directs its function, does not always allow one to remember the past. While the soul discards and effaces the memory of the extraneous details, it allows the distilled experiences to be stored in the depth of one's mind from life to life.

These are known as *saṃskāras*. The deepest memories, according to the *Yoga Sūtras* may take lifetimes to manifest. These are known as *vāsanās*.

Samskāric memory can be seen in the case of Mozart, where music of the spheres poured through his compositions even when he was a small child. Western science explained this as a mutation, whereas in India it is explained as gifts developed from *saṃskāras* or *vāsanās* of previous incarnations.

> *"You have come from bliss and no matter how deeply you get lost in the world, part of you remains in your blissful nature."*
>
> *-Sanatkumari*

SUPERNORMAL MEMORY

This part of memory is revelation or remembrance of one's Self, the essence of being. It is the higher intuitional memory of who and what we truly are. In this part of memory there is an awakening of our mind that will make ordinary consciousness seem like a state of sleep. It is the awakening of a memory that takes us to a greater awareness of joy, effectiveness and inner peace. It has been said that ordinary or normal consciousness is similar to a trancelike state in which the essential Self is suppressed and controlled by mechanical habits of thought, perception and behavior. When we awaken the supernormal memory from its dormant and sleeping state, we awaken vast areas of consciousness that are highly accessible to those seeking personal fulfillment and peace within themselves and the world.

This supernormal memory relates to *ānandamaya kośa*, or the auric sheath of bliss. It is the unveiling of the mysteries of the power of memory. The supernormal memory is connected with principles of hope, *prāṇic* energy, power of decisiveness, faith, conviction and ultimately, happiness. The supernormal memory cannot be limited by time, space and causation. It cannot be compared to any experience at all. It is not less or more, small or big, short-lived or long lasting.

Sanatkumari in Sage Narada's dialogue says, "You have come from bliss and no matter how deeply you get lost in the world, part of you remains in your blissful nature. It is that part which reminds you from within to search for and attain eternal boundless bliss and become one with it."

In supernormal memory, we hold the remembrance of our Divine nature. The urge to attain happiness is the driving force behind all pursuits in life. But, the charms and temptations of worldly objects are so strong that we forget to turn inwards and find the treasure of happiness that lies within ourselves. We miss that happiness that lies buried in the chamber of memory. To find it again, we may try to multiply our efforts to find happiness within the external world. We may work hard to attain material wealth or a beloved person in our life, thinking it will give us some degree of happiness and joy. But after a while, the happiness fades and we are dissatisfied again. Our senses dart outwards, looking for something or someone else. We continue our actions in the external world with the prime hope that the next attainment will bring happiness.

NOTE: A correlate of memory is fear. Fear can enter in to block supernormal memory; fear of not having enough, fear of losing what we already have accumulated. Fear, happiness, and bliss cannot coexist. If we do not have our own direct experience of superlative joy and bliss, we stand on trust of the experience of the saints and sages that have gone before us. It is that faith that gives the courage to seek the supernormal memory of bliss, not in our world but the hidden wealth that lies within us, of that deep memory of ānanda.

Memory in Buddhism
Supernormal memory is also paramount in the teaching of Buddhism and the path to enlightenment. In the story of Buddha's life, the night before his enlightenment at the zenith of his meditations, he remembered every single past life he had ever lived. The floodgates of the subconscious opened and a torrent of memories flooded his conscious mind. In the remembrance of every experience he had ever lived through, he saw *countless* past-lives lived in ignorance of truth. He realized the impermanence of this phenomenal experience and came to understand the cycle of impressions and reactions that keep the mind hurtling through lifetime after lifetime. This experience of total and complete memory recall is the last step before enlightenment and the cessation of the cycle of death and rebirth.

Another example of supernormal memory is from Dr. Haridas Chaudhuri who taught that supernormal memory is the remembrance of already being enlightened. "It is like my lost glasses. I can't see anything without them. I look everywhere for them. I've searched here and there. Finally, I stop. In exhaustion and a sense of futility, I bring my hand to my forehead. There they are, perched on the bridge of my nose! Ah hah," I exclaim, "Eureka! I have found them." Then his voice would drop. "But, did I ever lose them? They were there all the time while I was searching."

> *Supernormal memory is awakening to the vast knowledge that lies within the hidden depths of the psyche*

Supernormal memory is like the glasses, it is awakening to what already is. As our own search for 'truth' leads us upon many circuitous paths and eventually leads us back to where our feet stand. This search also leads back to the human heart where the nectar of immortality is stored. This coveted nectar is the knowledge that we are immortal and already one with our universal source. Supernormal memory is the remembrance that there is nowhere to go. We are already there.

MEMORY IN ĀSANA

In *yoga,* we see the body as crystallized mind, and we store every memory in every cell of the body. As the *sūtra* says, "memory is not allowing an object which has been experienced to escape." By not allowing that object to escape, each time you go into the posture you will try to recapture something delicious that you experienced before.

> *In yoga, we see the body as crystallized mind, we store every memory in every cell.*

If we can approach a pose as if we were practicing it for the very first time, our mind is fresh with care and attentiveness. When practicing the pose, we would keep our mind in the moment, not clinging to a positive experience from the past or projecting too far ahead with dread or anticipation. If we take the memory of how the body responded in the past and start afresh from that point our body can open even more, exploring ever-new depths within *āsana*. We are not trying to recapture past memories of the pose or revert to old familiar patterns.

When we are in the moment within the *āsana* and observe the memories that can arise from the storehouse of the subconscious mind, we begin to understand that *āsana* does not create, but reveals, what is already there. This is the practice of *smṛti sādhanā*.

EXERCISE:

Please Discuss or Journal on the Following Questions:

1) *Please briefly describe the three forms of smṛti, memory.*
2) *What are some positive and negative aspects of smṛti?*
3) *Have you observed abnormal memory in a friend or family member or in yourself? Can you relate this to psychological sleep, what yourself or others may want to "tune out"?*
4) *Have any memories ever surfaced during your practice of yoga? Please describe.*

HOW THE FIVE VṚTTIS OSCILLATE TOGETHER

Just as its difficult to know where the correct or accurate perception of *pramāṇa* slips into the distortion of the incorrect perception of *viparya*, it is difficult to separate incorrect perception and imagination. They alternate in their interaction with one another. The *vikalpa* or imagination also interacts with the dreamlike states in physical sleep and can distort the imagination in psychological sleep, which then has its impact on *smṛti* or memory. The order in which Patañjali has placed them is brilliant in its flow of logic and how one melts into the next.

The following is an example of how the five *vṛttis* interrelate and create turbulence within the mind. When the five non-painful mind waves are impacted by *ahaṁkāra* (ego), they can become painful. Instead of seeing others as our brother and sisters of the one humanity, our consciousness becomes separative and competitive. Instead of cooperation and collaboration in the workplace, a colleague may find a fact (*pramāṇa*) about a co-worker who is up for a promotion. In wanting that promotion for himself, the colleague discovers a fact about his teammate and negatively embellishes, exaggerates, and distorts the truth. He repeats it to others until they believe the rumor in their minds to be fact. The further it strays from the direct experience, into third- and fourth-hand information it becomes testimony or inference from others. People begin to believe it because they may not have a direct experience of the person who is being denigrated. This would be *viparyaya*, or incorrect perception. There is an old saying that pertains to the interweaving of *viparyaya* and *vikalpa,* "When a lie is repeated a hundred times, it becomes a truth."

The competitive teammate may eventually begin to believe the incorrect perception of the lies and propaganda, forgetting the origin of the truth (correct perception). His colleague is passed over for the promotion and he gets the position. By this time, his conscious mind believes the lies and distortions thinking them to be fact. He has gone to sleep (*nidrā*) as to what the truth is and feels justified in taking the position. As time passes, his memory becomes even more distorted and he thinks he was justified in his actions. He no longer knows what is truth or error. He cannot sleep and his health begins to suffer. There is a current in the deep and hidden recesses of his mind that knows the facts and that he has overreached and transgressed the boundaries of his own truth. In doing this, he has inflicted pain on another that can be seen as an act of violence. He has distorted the truth to achieve his own ends regardless of the hurt he has created for others. This undertow in his conscience distorts his memory and he is in pain, having forgotten its origins. His work is affected and he is soon fired from the company.

Another example would be how CEO John Scully, hired by Steve Jobs, eventually manipulated the board of Apple into firing Steve Jobs, the visionary and founder, forcing him to leave the very company that he had founded.

From the interaction of the five *vṛttis* (*pramāṇa, viparyaya, vikalpa, nidrā* and *smṛti*), and their interaction with the four parts of mind (*manas, ahaṁkāra, citta* and *buddhi*) an experience is created. These accumulated experiences determine how we perceive life. The *vṛttis* arise out of the *citta* and lead to desire; that desire leads us to taking an action (*karma*) to fulfill the desire; that action leads us to an experience; and the experience leads to the formulation of a subconscious impression (*saṃskāra*). That *saṃskāra* embeds itself within the psyche. When it bubbles up again it comes as a new *vṛtti*, which means *to rise upwards and come into existence.* And the cycle begins again (see the "wheel of cause and effect" chart in Chapter II).

This entire cycle can be halted at the point of the *vṛttis.* If one can observe, understand and exercise mastery over these five *vṛttis* or waves of the mind, they can actually become constructive instead of destructive. When the *ahaṁkāra*, ego, is not involved in making these non-painful *vṛttis* painful, then we no longer need the *yamas* and *niyamas* in the eight limbs of *yoga* to reverse the affects of the *vṛttis* and *kleśas* (painful *vṛttis*) and dissolve the *saṃskāras* back into their original source. If we can master this piece of the *vṛttis*, we can negate the entire cycle of cause and effect. We can then enter the state of *yogaś citta vṛtti nirodaḥ* and we need not move into the second chapter of the *Yoga Sūtras.*

EXERCISE:

Write an evaluation of how the vṛttis manifest in your life:

1. *Observe and describe the three parts of pramāṇa vṛtti and how it is operating in your life and how it can easily lead to viparyaya.*
2. *Give at least one example of how the interaction of viparyaya and vikalpa (incorrect perception and imagination) has led to conflict and confusion in your life.*
3. *What is the source or cause of expectation based upon the five non-painful vṛttis*
4. *When you don't feel heard, valued and honored for who you are, where is the source?*
5. *If you do not feel "heard," are you listening? Evaluate and discuss.*
6. *What are the emotions of not being heard that arise out of the thought waves?*
7. *Smṛti (memory) has three parts:*
    a. *abnormal memory, forgetfulness, amnesia, dementia, or alzheimer's;*
    b. *normal memory, remembrance of what we have learned so far in our life, normal activities; and*
    c. *supernormal memory, remembering our "at-one-ness" with others and our existing connection with the universal source.*

    Please observe, write and discuss how these three parts of memory can possibly be operable simultaneously.
8. *How Does nidrā impact memory?*
9. *Please give at least one example of how these five vṛttis are operating in your life at this time.*
10. *Call to mind a person who has caused you pain or discomfort in some fashion. Write about the ways in which you are similar to this person.*

HOMEPLAY: *For the next 2 weeks, observe the interplay of the five vrittis in all your life's activities.*

I.12 ABHYĀSA VAIRĀGYĀBHYĀṂ TANNIRODHAḤ

Abhyāsa *= 'a' is to reverse and 'bhyasa' means outward or downward pull. This is commonly translated as continual practice.*
Vairāgya *= 'vi' to negate and 'ragya' comes from 'rāga' which means mood. This means non-mood or non-attachment.*
Abhyam *= by both*
Tan *= from 'tad' which means going beyond self-imposed limitations*
Nirodaḥ *= restrained, quiet, still, calm*

I translate this *sūtra* as:
We 'Go Beyond,' Using Continual Practice And Non-attachment To Quiet And Still The Waves Of The Mind.

Translations are usually:
By (Continual) Practice And Non-attachment, (Mind Waves) Can Be Tranquil And Still.
We Can Still The Vṛttis Through Continual Practice And Non-attachment.

ABHYĀSA

The short *a* means to reverse and *bhaya* is outward or downward. *Abhyāsa* literally means to reverse or check the downward pull. This is the first word Patañjali gives in the *Yoga Sūtras* as a way to still the waves of the mind (*tan nirodaḥ*). Even though *abhyāsa* literally is "to check the downward pull" it is usually defined as continual and uninterrupted practice. Obviously, the continual practice would be "checking the downward pull" not only of body, but also of mind and emotions. It is continual self observation as well as rising above the downward pull that can arise in life's situations.

VAIRĀGYA

The prefix *vi* means to reverse and *rāga* is mood or passion commonly referred to as "attachment." *Vairāgya* then is defined as detachment, non-attachment or dispassion. The English derivative of the Sanskrit *rāga* is rage and sometimes referred to as passion. If the object of our affection or attachment is no longer available to us, our emotions based on passion can turn into aversion, anger and rage.

In the state of *vairāgya*, a *yogin* is neutral between attachment and aversion, *rāga* and *dveṣa*, praise or blame, criticism or compliments. The polarities that pull our minds in one direction and then another, creating mental turbulence and restlessness, have an opportunity to come into balance through *vairāgya*.

Abhyāsa and *vairāgya* are a form of *jñāna yoga* or the *yoga* of wisdom. *Jñāna yoga* is based upon discrimination, discernment, dedication and even devotion. In this *sūtra, abhyāsa* and *vairāgya* require constant and continual vigilance. In *jñāna yoga* we transform the intellect into higher intuition through holding the mind in the remembrance that we are already one with the universal source. In this *sūtra,* the continual practice would be holding the mind in that state of remembrance and non-attachment.

> *Love Plus Detachment Equals Compassion*
>
> *-Dalai Llama*

TAN NIRODAḤ

Tan Nirodah is the thinning of the *kleśas* (painful mindwaves) and quieting of the waves of the mind. *Tan* means "going beyond self-imposed limitations." It is an intensive stretch that takes us beyond limitations to a point of self-transformation. *Ni* is to negate and *rodaḥ* is from *Rudra*, the Vedic god of storms. When there are storms there is howling and turbulence. The mind cannot come to rest. It is even difficult to sleep at night when there is thunder, lightening and a deluge of rain. *Nirodaḥ* would mean to calm and quiet the storms and turbulence of the mind. These two words together would mean, "to go beyond past limitations to quiet the fluctuations that arise within the field of the mind."

IN ĀSANA

In the practice of *āsana*, we release habitually contracted muscles before we can come into the place of stillness where relaxation takes place. As space is created within our body, we also create space within the mind by gradually increasing space between each thought. This brings both body and mind into ever deepening states of relaxation and stillness.

The word *tan* is found in names of many *āsanas* such as *Uttānāsana*, *Paścimottanāsana*, and *Pūrvotānāsana*. In these *āsanas* the midline of the body is lengthened and thinned. *Tan* is an intensive stretch that takes us beyond past limitations in our cellular structure into an evolutionary spiral of self-transformation. *Tan* is a form of *abhyāsa*, "checking the downward pull" of past contractions that have compressed inner space weighing us down physically, mentally and emotionally.

Tan nirodaḥ can be practiced in *āsana* with each exhalation as we elongate the spine to create growing space within the internal organs. This also creates space within the mind bringing both body and mind into gradual equilibrium and deepening states of relaxation and stillness.

By creating inner space within our inner organs, we can experience a growing lightness and sense of freedom. One of the subtle benefits of *yoga* is to release *saṃskāras*, the cellular memories stored within the psyche, to bring them up for releasing and healing. In this particular *sutra*, Patañjali is saying that it is through *abhyāsa* and *vairāgya* one can come into that state of *tan nirodaḥ*, the stillness of mind.

> *May I be shown the non-oscillating state of dynamic fullness as I empty myself of the fetters of attachment*

I.13 TATRA STHITAU YATNO 'BHYĀSAḤ

Tatra = *of these*
Sthitau = *in steadiness*
Yatnaḥ = *effort*
Abhyāsaḥ = *practice*

Of These Two, Effort Toward Steadiness Of Mind Is Practice.

This *sūtra* moves deeper into the concept of *abhyāsa*, or continual practice. The attainment of *abhyāsa* is through effort (*yatnaḥ*) and steadiness (*sthiti*).

YATNAḤ – EFFORT
What is meant by effort? When we speak of the steadiness of effort, this does not mean implementing external force upon the mind, which results in more mental and physical tension, but comes from a deep internal source of energy. To relax this external effort requires faith and offering to a power that is greater than one's self. The self-will offers itself to a higher will. When we can go into the deepest place within our self, we are able to relax the effort that manifests in the outer body. We can then come from that unseen strength that lies deep within our spiritual core.

Here the word effort does not mean pushing, straining or exerting one's ego in striving. This type of effort would be described in the *Bhagavad Gītā* as, "the inaction within the action." It would be described in Buddhism as "Right Effort," which is a great friend and tool to surmount obstacles in the path towards enlightenment. Notice they make a distinction between *effort* and *Right Effort,* which is in fact the 'art of doing nothing.' It is the effort required to draw the mind back to its state of equilibrium and then surrender the effort. A tense and contracted effort, that is striving or forcing, produces tension and exhaustion and becomes detrimental to attaining a relaxed equilibrium of mind.

YATNAḤ, EFFORT, WITHIN ĀSANA

> *Through Relaxation of Effort and Meditation Upon the Infinite, Asana is Perfected*
>
> *Sutra II:37*

In *āsana*, this means not muscling through the postures, which causes more physical tension and grasping of the mind. In *āsana*, if the spine is *rajasic*, the head is *tamasic* (in relaxation) the pose becomes *sattvic*; there is no effort from the mind. In the pose, *Utthita Padotānāsana*, one lies on the back and lowers the legs from a 90-degree angle to the floor. The common impulse is to use the rectus abdominis muscles and puff out the abdomen to achieve the strength to lower the legs with control. In fact, in Western anatomy and physiology, they say this is the only way to lower the legs. Through the teachings of *yoga*, we find the strength that lies much deeper than the rectus abdominis muscles and only through the relaxation of those muscles can we find the deeper strength, the true core strength, in this *āsana*. In lifting or lowering the legs it comes from a source other than our musculature. The mind is relaxed, the spinal cord is active and elongated and the pose is *sattvic*. It is surrender of the musculature of the mind that finds the place where the musculature of the body can find a deeper strength, found only through the release of tension. *Āsana* is a wonderful way to practice the "relaxation of effort through meditation upon the infinite."

STITHI – STEADINESS

The *sūtras* tell us that the "practice of a*bhyāsa* is the acquiring of a tranquil mind (*sthiti*) which is the absence of fluctuations or undisturbed calmness." *Sthiti* is from *stha*, which means to establish steadiness or unwavering immovability. *Sthiti* is that outflow that comes out of *stha*, it is the same as the flow of virtue we want to cultivate. When the *citta* of the mind is without *vṛttis*, it flows in a calm state. That is *sthiti*, which means perfection, being fixed and established in a stage or state. *Stithi* doesn't mean flow itself, it means being perfected in that state. Like a tightrope walker moving toward the other end of the rope, they are established in steadiness and concentration to maintain their balance.

In *sthiti* the *rajas* and *tamas guṇas* are not functioning and the flow is toward the *sattvic* state of mind. *Sattva* is the original state of the mind. *Rajas* and *tamas* are the forces that work upon the mind to pull it out of *sthiti* and its established equilibrium. *Sthiti* is the return to the original state of the mind that is stable and unwavering, free from restlessness (*rajas*) and dull lethargy (*tamas*). When the three *guṇas* are in balance it is known as *Ātma sthiti*, or '*sthiti* of the soul.'

Note: For More Information on the Gunas refer to the Guna Box (pg. VIII)

I.14 SA TU DĪRGHA KĀLA NAIRANTARYA SATKĀRĀSEVITO DṚḌHABHŪMIḤ

Sa *= this*
Tu *= and*
Dīrgha *= long*
Kāla *= time*
Nairantarya *= without break, continuous*
Satkāra *= earnestness*
Asevito *= well attended to*
Dṛḍha *= firm*
Bhūmiḥ *= ground*

Practice Becomes Firmly Grounded When Well Attended To For A Long Time, Without Break And In All Earnestness.

When *sthiti* is established in *abhyāsa*, our practice is not broken or interrupted by a habit of restlessness, it is considered to be continual practice. Continuous practice is constant self-observation and reflection, as well as carrying that into the practice of *āsana*, *prāṇāyāma* and *dhyāna*. It is the continual refinement of our own practice of *yamas* and *niyamas*, the ten commandments of *yoga* (see II:30 to II:45).

To persevere with a continual practice, according to *sūtra* commentaries, requires unwavering faith, enthusiasm, stamina and energy (*vīrya*). The Muṇḍaka Upaniṣad says, "This self is realized not by one who has no energy, nor by one who is subject to delusion, nor by knowledge." It is believed that when a wise *yogin* establishes a continuity of practice, the soul reaches the abode of "Brahman," the universal consciousness.

Sūtras I:13 and I:14 explore the concept of *abhyāsa* more deeply from I:12. Here we will expound and explore *abhyāsa*, the concept of 'continual practice' or as I define it, 'checking the downward pull' within *āsana*.

ABHYĀSA IN ĀSANA

Abhyāsa is an amazing concept to practice in *āsana*. *Abhyāsa* could be considered to be the gravitational pull on our emotions and mind. It also refers to the downward pull of our bodies. The mind is reflected in our body's posture.

One of ways we can check the downward pull according to scripture, is through devotion. Devotion is considered to be an offering of one's self to the universal. Throughout the *Yoga Sūtras* there are references of *samādhi* coming quickly to those who are devoted and surrender to *Īśvara*, the Lord of this world, the teacher of even the most ancients (see I:23 through I:28).

Āsanas are conscious movements representing our life's actions and can be practiced as offerings to the Divine. In every *āsana*, it is important to remember *abhyāsa* and continually practice lifting above the downward gravitational field that manifests as compression in our body as well as depression in the mind. We can practice *abhyāsa* in *āsana* through the elongation of the spine on each exhalation. The body has a tendency to sink into itself when we breathe out. However, if we were to do the opposite and rise up out of ourselves on the out-breath, even negative thought patterns can lift above their usual downward pull.

> *In every asana, it is important to remember abhyāsa and continually practice lifting above the downward gravitational field that manifests as compression in our body as well as depression in the mind.*

In *abhyāsa* if we can grow down through the part of the body that is closer to the earth, this becomes the force or leverage to lengthen the spine and lift out of the gravitational pull. In honoring both polarities, we offer to the earth and the heavens simultaneously. If we are creating a triangular base in headstand, we offer our forearms and inner elbows to the earth and the soles of the feet to the heavens. In *yoga*, the head is the seat of ego, and in headstand it is humbled to the earth. In shoulderstand, we humble the head to the heart and the outer edges of the elbows and outer scapula to the earth, as the seventh cervical vertebra and the entire spine rises upward in *abhyāsa*.

Inverted poses check the downward pull and also create a different spatial relationship, helping one to overcome fear by practicing a new variation that represents the unknown. The head in *yoga* represents the ego. The heart is above the head in both headstand and shoulderstand and the heart becomes supreme over the ego. Through the practice of *abhyāsa* in these poses, the ego has an opportunity to lift itself into the light and expansion of the *buddhi* consciousness.

In *Tadāsana*, our feet have an opportunity to give a devotional offering to the earth as we lift the inner arch as the ball of the big toe and circumference of the heels grow down into the earth like the roots of a great tree. To practice *abhyāsa* in *āsana*, we use gravity to transcend gravity. As the knees lift upwards, away from the gravitational field, it strengthens and lifts the pelvic organs preventing prolapse. As the base of the tailbone and buttocks move down toward the earth, the rest of the spine rises upward out of the pelvic basin. As the shoulders drop down away from the ears, the heart center offers itself upward. As the neck lengthens, drawing the ears away from the shoulders, it is all *abhyāsa*, checking the downward pull by using gravity to transcend itself.

Abhyāsa can be practiced in every *āsana* as torso and limbs are lifted and elongated. It can be practiced in life by lifting and lengthening our spine instead of slouching in our chairs, car seats or even standing and walking. When we walk there is a tendency for our mind to drop down as the forward foot touches the earth. This can create spinal compression. What would happen if you were to lift up out of yourself each time your feet embrace the earth? In this way, we can extend and transcend the gravitational pull of the earth, while connecting to it.

To practice *abhyāsa* in the meditative seat, as the back thighs grow down into the earth, the spine rises up. As the skin of the back rolls down on the exhalation, the front of the sternum rises in remembrance and devotion to the Divine.

Even the breath is an aspect of *abhyāsa*. On the exhalation, instead of sinking into ourselves, if we "check the downward pull" and rise up out of ourselves as we move into a pose, it is *abhyāsa*. In the practice of *abhyāsa*, one part of the body offers itself to the earth as another part offers to the heavens. This bilateral integration of *āsana* uses the body as a vehicle for self-transformation.

In the practice of abhyāsa, one part of the body offers itself to the earth as another part offers to the heavens. This bilateral integration of āsana uses the body as a vehicle for self-transformation.

Even our posture can reflect the *buddhi* state of consciousness as well as *abhyāsa* in all situations in our life especially when we want to revert back to old patterns that don't serve us anymore. This could relate to any type of addiction or people who are not a positive influence in our life. As we transcend past patterns through *abhyāsa*, we can eventually transform and transform ego into the *buddhi* consciousness.

One morning, while Mr. B.K.S. Iyengar was staying in my home in California, a neighbor came over complaining of fatigue and depression. Mr. Iyengar looked at her compressed posture. Her shoulders were rounded, her head hung forward and her spine was collapsing. He said, "Madam, lift your sternum, elongate your neck, roll your shoulders back, open your armpits to the sky." Suddenly, she was in *Tadāsana*, where the crown of her head was aligned with the base of the spine. Her shoulders were open, her spine elongated and her heart center was lifting to the light of the morning sun. "Oh, I feel so different, I feel so good, I feel wonderful—what did you do?" Her eyes were bright, she was smiling and when she began to walk away, her step was buoyant. Mr. Iyengar shook his head sadly and said, "I don't know which comes first...compression or depression."

When he aligned her pose in *abhyāsa*, he checked the downward pull of not just her body but of her mind and emotions. This was a wonderful learning experience of how compression of the body can often lead to depression of the mind and how depression can lead to compression.

I.15 DṚṢṬĀNUŚRAVIKA VIṢAYA VITṚṢNASYA VAŚĪKĀRA SAṂJÑĀ VAIRĀGYAM

Dṛṣṭa *= seen, experienced*
Anuśravika *= heard, revealed*
Viṣaya *= object*
Vitṛṣnasya *= of him who is free from cravings*
Vaśīkāra *= mastery*
Saṃjña *= consciousness, clear knowledge*
Vairāgyam *= non-attachment*

The Consciousness Of Self-mastery In One Who Is Free From Craving Objects (Seen Or Heard About) Is Non-attachment.

I came across a very old commentary on the *sūtras* that says, "There is nothing wrong with attachment, only the need to repeat it." Attachments are considered to have a repetitive nature. We want to repeat whatever gives us sweetness or pleasure. This obviously relates to desires that can lead to cravings and in turn addictions that contribute more turbulence within the mind. Sigmund Freud, the father of Western psychology discovered what Eastern *yogi's* have known for thousands of years. If a desire is unfilled, it becomes a craving. The craving propels us into an action to satisfy itself. When we go to great lengths to fulfill our cravings, it is not so much to achieve the object of our desire but to relax the tension that the craving produces.

Yoga Sūtra 1:37 commentaries say that "if one's own mind can be freed from desires, and thus free from thoughts, and if that state of the mind can be mastered by practice, then also the mind becomes free from attachment to objects. This is the practice of non-attachment."

Non-attachment means demanding nothing for the separative soul. In this state, everything will come effortlessly. If we can free ourselves from the clinging chains of attachment, we can achieve true freedom. Freedom, in this context, does not mean necessarily leaving a situation, but transforming our attitude towards that situation.

There is a very thin line between detachment and indifference. Sometimes we think we are unattached, when we are indifferent to a situation or person. The yogis have said we cannot know detachment until we have first known attachment.

Detachment would not mean self and societal protection or aloofness and withdrawal. Instead, we could view the deeper elements of detachment as seeing all people truly as they are. If we look deep enough into what we perceive as the faults of others, we can see their virtue, divinity and humanity, and the one light that shines in all. Detachment accesses the *buddhi* mind, which is the onlooker to all that occurs.

Baba Haridas defines this *sūtra* as, "When mind loses all desire for objects seen and unseen, it acquires a state of utter desirelessness known as detachment." He speaks of attaining this state of *vairāgya* through four stages:

1. YATAMĀNA

In *yatamāna* one continually observes attachments and aversions (*rāga* and *dveṣa*) of the senses. Through continuous observation and attempting to reduce indulgences, attachments and aversions lessen their hold over the senses. (see II:7 and II:8 for more on *rāga* and *dveṣa*)

2. VYATIREKA

Vyatireka is a state of dispassion where some attachments of the senses have been eliminated and others may remain but the link is feeble. Contact with objects of cravings and aversions become lessened and as a result the senses can begin to withdraw towards the center of one's being.

3. EKENDRIYA

Eka means one and *indriya* are senses. This means *ekendriya* is 'one sense' which can be the integration of the five senses. It is the state where all attachments and aversions are weaned from the senses and the senses resolve into the mind. The attachment that remains exists within the mind and not the senses. (This can be compared with *pratyāhāra* in the second chapter, II:54 and II:55.) In *ekendriya*, the *prāṇa* or life force resides within the mind and does not move out through the senses. But if one continues to interact with the objects of the senses, the mind can be pulled back to attachment.

4. VAŚIKĀRA

Vaśikāra is the state where all attachments and aversions are wiped clean from the mind, and desire and aversion cease. The senses and the mind have pulled into the center of being, it demands nothing for itself, it is able to be the onlooker to all that occurs and practice true compassion (love with detachment). The state of *Vaśikāra* is not reached at once and is attained through the previous three stages. *Vaśikāra* is also called *aparavairāgya*, which eventually moves into *paravairāgya*, which means 'supreme detachment.' It is the most expanded state of *vairāgya*.

Now, how can we apply this to the practice of *āsana*?

VAIRĀGYA IN ĀSANA

When we release attachments to a desired result in *āsana*, it is the practice of *vairāgya*. The neutrality of *vairāgya* can be practiced in *āsana* by expanding consciousness equally into every part of the body, not overextending one area while holding resistance in another. *Vairāgya* is the transcendence of desires. It would reflect in *āsana* by only going to our 'edge' not over-reaching, striving or competing with others not even with ourselves. If we were to practice *āsana* as a "*vairāgi*," we would not strive to attain a goal. We would do our practice not to get somewhere or something from it...but to do the practice for its sake alone.

We can practice *vairāgya* by being neutral and equanimous in the center of postural attachments and aversions, or between feelings of success or failure in a pose. As a *vairāgi*, we would practice the more difficult and challenging poses as well as those that bring pleasure and comfort. We would accept all with equal ease, staying in our *svādharma* (what is right for us) releasing emotional resistance as well as excessive attachment to a goal knowing that everything we desire is already within us. *Yoga Sūtra* commentaries say that, "Detachment is the culmination of knowledge. *Kaivalya* (liberation) and detachment are inseparable."

Accept all postures with equal ease, staying in your svādharma, release emotional resistance as well as excessive attachment to a goal knowing that everything you desire is already within you.

EXERCISE:

Please Discuss or Journal on the Following Questions:

1) *How would you apply abhyāsa to your yoga practice? To your life?*
2) *Thinking of some situations in your life, which have you succeeded in applying vairāgya and which have you not?*
3) *In what areas of your life are you putting forth yatnaḥ? Is this creating tension? Are you able to find 'right effort' or the 'inaction within the action'?*

HOMEPLAY: *For the next 2 weeks, apply the principles of abhyāsa, yatnaḥ and sthithi within your āsana practice. Can you find the place where āsana is perfected through the relaxation of effort and meditation upon the infinite?*

I.16 TAT PARAṂ PURUṢA KHYĀTER GUṆAVAITṚṢṆYAM

Tat *= that*
Paraṃ *= supreme*
Puruṣa *= true self*
Khyāter *= due to the realization*
Guṇa *= of any of the constituents of nature*
Vaitṛṣṇyam *= non-thirst*

Indifference To The *Guṇas*, The Constituent Principles, Achieved Through Knowledge Of The Nature Of *Puruṣa* Is Called *Para-vairāgya* (Supreme Detachment).

This is a very exciting *sūtra* because it clarifies and helps define *asmitā* (egoism) that is the second of the five painful mind-waves known as *kleśas* as mentioned in II:6. "Egoism mistakenly identifies the power of the seer, *puruṣa,* with that of the seen which is the *buddhi.*" It is amazing to see here in this *sūtra* that if an aspirant practices detachment and achieves the supreme or ultimate state of detachment known as *para-vairāgya*, they will know *puruṣa* (the substratum of Being). According to this *sūtra,* supreme detachment is the culmination of knowledge and *kaivalya* (liberation). They are considered inseparable.

This is the first *sūtra* where Patañjali mentions the *guṇas*. There are three *guṇas*. They are: l) *sattva* 2) *rajas* and 3) *tamas*. The *guṇas* are responsible for the mental modifications or *vṛttis* that arise within the field of the mind (*citta*). *Gund* means to bind. The *guṇas* are the constituents that bind and give form to matter. They are magnetic forces that keep our world on its axis.

The three *guṇas* are electromagnetic fields that give rise to the fluctuations of the *vṛttis* (mind waves). At times, one *guṇa* is more prominent than another. It is their interactive modulations that create life as well as oscillations in the human mind, thoughts and emotions.

1) *Rajas guṇa* manifests as activity, restlessness, and mobility
2) *Sattva guṇa* manifests as a sense of lightness, peacefulness, serenity and equanimity.
3) *Tamas guṇa* is inert, heavy, lethargic, and immobile.

Which *guṇa* is more active determines the quality of our thoughts when they arise. One may predominate over the other but through *yoga*, they can be brought into balance. All of *yoga* is meant to create equilibrium of these three *guṇas*. When the *guṇas* come into balance, the mind becomes still within the state of *Yogaś Citta Vṛtti Nirodhaḥ*.

All of yoga is meant to create equilibrium of these three guṇas [sattva, rajas and tamas]. When the guṇas come into balance, the mind becomes still within the state of Yogaś Citta Vṛtti Nirodhaḥ

This *sūtra* also mentions, "Indifference to the *guṇas*." What does this mean? Indifference in *yoga* usually means neutrality. In that state of indifference, it's like being in the *buddhi* mind centered in the midst of all polarities and perspectives. It is a form of *paravairāgya* or supreme detachment. In this state, the oscillating fluctuations of the *guṇas* have no hold over our mind; they come into perfect equilibrium, and stillness. This is *Yogaś Citta Vṛtti Nirodhaḥ*.

In regard to the Supreme Detachment of *paravairāgya*, the *Kaṭha Upaniṣad* says, "The wise, knowing of the eternal bliss, do not look for the immutable in ephemeral things."

Note: It is interesting to observe at each interval of this first chapter that Patañjali gives many ways for the aspirant to realize God but they seem to be more challenging and less concrete than the verses in the second chapter. Could it be that this chapter is meant for the more intense or sattvic student of yoga?

I.17 VITARKA VICĀRĀNANDĀSMITĀNUGAMĀT SAṂPRAJÑĀTAḤ

Vitarka *= reasoning*
Vicāra *= reflecting*
Ānanda *= rejoicing*
Asmitā *= pure I-am-ness*
Anugamāt *= due to the following, from accompaniment*
Saṃprajñātaḥ *= distinguishing, discerning (Samādhi – contemplation)*

When Concentration Is Reached With The Help Of *Vitarka, Vicāra, Ānanda* and *Asmitā*, It Is Called *Saṃprajñāta Samādhi*.

Saṃprajñāta comes out of *saṃ* which is bringing it all together in the sum total or to become one with, *pra* to bring forth and *jñāta* is from *jñāna* which means knowledge or wisdom. So *saṃprajñāta samādhi* is "becoming one with and bringing forth the wisdom." With wisdom, an aspirant is said to find discernment.

Saṃprajñāta samādhi is where the fluctuations of the waves of the mind have been quieted or stilled through "practice and detachment" (*abhyāsa* and *vairāgya*). These are addressed in previous *sūtras* (1:12 through 1:16). Usually this state is known as an "arrested" state of mind. I don't usually use this term, as it sounds a bit officious and repressive. However, in *saṃprajñāta samādhi*, the mind is not fully "arrested," but is considered to be in a partially arrested state. This form of *samādhi* is realized through a mind that is habitually one-pointed.

Saṃprajñāta Samādhi is the form of realized consciousness that still holds the seeds of manifestation or afflictions (*kleśas*) from past actions and experience. This means that the seeds of worldly consciousness are still in the *citta*. In this state of *samādhi* there are still fluctuations of the *vṛttis* (mind waves) and the seeds of past experiences are still embedded in the psyche. With the right opportunity, these seeds can germinate again. This would keep the mind in what may be considered a "lower" state of *samādhi* that can lead to birth, death and rebirth.

> *Saṃprajñāta samādhi is,*
> *'becoming one with and bringing forth the wisdom'*

In this *sūtra*, when Patañjali says that *saṃprajñātaḥ samādhi* can be reached with the help of 1) *vitarka* 2) *vicāra* 3) *ānanda* and 4) *asmitā*, the *sūtra* unravels into greater complexity.

1) *Vitarka*, reasoning, is when the concentrated mind is filled with the gross (more physical) form of perceptions and realizes them.

2) *Vicāra* concentration relates to subtle objects. *Vicāra* is reflection. It is an aspect of *nirbīja samādhi*. *Nir* means not or without and *bīja* means seed. *Vicāra* is without seed where the seeds of afflictions (*kleśas*) have been scorched and will not multiply into future *vṛttis*. *Vicāra* refers to subtle objects and a feeling of felicity or happiness. This can be experienced through concentration of the breath. Concentration on bliss is free from *vitarka* and *vicāra*. It is an experiential understanding.

3) *Ānanda,* is the next word Patañjali gives for helping to attain the experience of *saṃprajñāta samādhi*. *Ānanda* is a feeling of felicity, a blissful sensation that is felt in the mind as well as in every cell of one's being. Concentration on bliss is free from *vitarka* and *vicāra*. It is beyond concentration on gross or subtle things.

4) *Asmitā* is the next word Patañjali gives to help bring forth *Saṃprajñāta Samādhi*. *Asmitā,* refers in this chapter, to the "I-Sense" or awareness of the individual personality.

This is very interesting because later in II:6, Patañjali speaks of transcending *asmitā,* which is one of the "five painful mind waves" known as *kleśas*. *Asmitā* confuses *buddhi* with *puruṣa*. It is a form of misconception on a grander scale, confusing the temporal for the eternal.

Eloquently, Swami Hariharānanda discusses in his commentary, "the subtle connection between the *puruṣa* and *buddhi* and when that is eliminated through *viveka-khyāti* (light of discrimination), *buddhi* disappears." This is quite wonderful, because in *asmitā*, (egoism) one would think that *buddhi,* which is the reflection of *puruṣa*, is actually *puruṣa* itself.

In the various samādhi states, we feel the magnetic pull of God where we no longer feel bound only by the gravitational pull of earth. In this state, we are like the lotus, rooted to the earth while floating lightly above the waters of life.

Asmitā mātrā is the pure "I-sense" that is free from even the sense of bliss. *Asmitā* is the innermost center of the mind that holds all parts of mind together. The mind plays a creative part in the universe. Knowledge is the result of interaction between the mind and the senses.

Swami Hariharānanda Āraṇya is brilliant in his commentaries on this *sūtra*, giving the many lesser-known stages that one enters into before entering into the more known stages of *samādhi*. These are:

1) *Savitarkā samādhi* is cognitive concentration on the gross form, such as the visible shape of a deity.
2) *Savicāra samādhi* is ecstasy with form. Attention is focused on the subtle object or the energy of the form. For example, to meditate "with feeling," on the form of a deity or something inspirational is *savicāra*.
3) *Sānanda samādhi* (*sa* means with and *ānanda* is bliss, *sānanda* then means with bliss). Since *samādhi* is defined as "to become one with," the state of *sānanda samādhi* would be the immersion of consciousness into the feeling sensation of profound joy and bliss.

The varying *samādhi* states are referred to as being in the uppermost center in the crown of the head. It is known as *sahasrāra* or "thousand-petaled lotus." Even though the lotus is connected by its stalk to the earth beneath the water, the flower floats lightly upon the surface opening and closing to the light of the morning and evening sun. This most beautiful of flowers grows from the mud beneath. It does not absorb the mud or water and does not "drown" but floats lightly above the water where even tiny droplets cannot penetrate the surface of its petals. The lotus flower is a symbol of the "One" who lives in the innermost center of our being without being drowned. It is a beautiful symbol of how the varying stages of *samādhi* lift our consciousness like the lotus flower, from the darkness from which it grows, upward to receive the light of universal consciousness.

The lotus is also a pose for meditation that recycles energy back into the spine bringing the *prāṇa* into the uppermost region of the head. In the meditative seat, *prāṇa* from the peripheral *nāḍīs* of the subtle body are gathered at the base of the stalk of the spine (coccyx and sacrum) that is the storehouse of the *kuṇḍalinī śakti*. This ancient powerful energy that dates back to the beginning of time, is also known in our modern world as bio-nuclear or psycho-nuclear energy. When it awakens, it reveals the stored microcosmic energy that is the reflection of the universal macrocosm. In the various *samādhi* states we feel the magnetic pull of God, where we no longer feel bound only by the gravitational pull of earth. In this state, we are like the lotus, rooted to the earth while floating lightly above the waters of life.

The lotus flower is a symbol of the "One" who lives in the innermost center of our being without being drowned. It is a beautiful symbol of how the varying stages of samādhi lift our consciousness like the lotus flower, from the darkness from which it grows, upward to receive the light of universal consciousness.

I.18 VIRĀMA PRATYAYĀBHYĀSA PŪRVAḤ SAṂSKĀRAŚEṢO'NYAḤ

Virāma *= complete cessation*
Pratyaya *= content of mind*
Abhyāsa *= by the practice*
Pūrvaḥ *= of the previous*
Saṁskāra *= impressions*
Śeṣaḥ *= remain*
Anyaḥ *= the other (Samādhi)*

Asaṃprajñāta Samādhi Is The Other Kind Of *Samādhi* That Arises Through Constant Practice Of *Paravairāgya*, Which Brings About The Disappearance Of All Fluctuations Of The Mind.

The previous *sūtra* discusses *saṃprajñāta samādhi* where the mind fluctuations still exist in a minute form and therefore contribute to the souls return to this world of *prakṛti*. *Asaṃprajñāta samādhi* on the other hand is the state of "seedless *samādhi*" where the seeds of affliction are scorched and cannot germinate again even when conditions are ripe. According to Patañjali, this particular *samādhi* is achieved through constant practice of *paravairāgya* defined as "supreme non-attachment."

> *Asaṃprajñāta Samādhi is the state of "seedless samādhi," where the seeds of affliction are scorched and cannot germinate again even when conditions are ripe.*

Para means beyond, *vi* means to negate and *rāga* is mood, from which the English word rage is derived. In *paravairāgya*, which is the supreme or highest state of "non-mood" or "non-attachment," the waves of the mind are calm and unwavering and free from craving. In the state of *paravairāgya*, there are no attachments and the seeds of afflictions (*kleśas*) sewn by attachments (*rāga*) are burnt never to arise or sprout again. *Paravairāgya* creates a *nirbīja* (seedless) or objectiveless *samādhi* that is *asaṃprajñāta samādhi*.

Asaṃprajñāta samādhi is an egoless state beyond the need of objects of concentration and beyond desires for any worldly objects. In *asaṃprajñāta samādhi* the soul is liberated and free from the rounds of birth, span of life and experiences (see II:13 and II:14).

Sage Vaśiṣṭha teaches Lord Rama on the glory of supreme detachment, "All that is painful is caused by attachment alone. Oh Rama, the mind should not be allowed to be attached to enjoyments, to actions, to the worries of the past, to the objects of the present, to the sky above, nor to the earth below, neither should it be attached to any of the four directions, nor to anything in between."

The great Sage Vaśiṣṭha also reminded Rama to not even allow the mind to be attached to any part of the body, whether it be the center between the eyebrows, the palate, the eye-balls, the mouth, or the *cakra* centers of the *kuṇḍalinī*. It is this type of supreme detachment (*paravairāgya*) that leads to the highest and most expansive form of *asaṃprajñāta samādhi*.

I.19 BHAVAPRATYAYO VIDEHA PRAKṚTILAYĀNĀM

Bhava *= existence, birth*
Pratyayaḥ *= content of mind (mental modification)*
Videha *= bodiless (Gods and spirits)*
Prakṛtilayānām *= merged into nature*

Those Who Merely Leave Their Physical Bodies And Attain The State Of Celestial Deities, (Bodiless Gods And Spirits) Who Get Merged In Nature, (*Prakṛtilayā*) Have Rebirth.

In this *sūtra*, *videhas*, the discarnate *devas* who are the "shining ones," live in a state that is like *kaivalya* (the state of liberation) with a mind functioning only as far as the radius of their latent impressions will allow. *Videhas* are divine disembodied beings known as the discarnate ones who have not realized the supreme *puruṣa*. It seems as if even these celestial beings known as *devas* carry within them the germ of *adarśana*. The short *a* reverses and *darśan* from *dṛṣ* meaning to see, therefore *adarśana* is not seeing. In this *sūtra* it would imply that even the *videhas*, the discarnate *devas* are not "really" seeing and they are not fully aware of the ultimate truth. Thus, when the time arises, they will be born again (*prakṛtilayānām*). *Prakṛti* means nature and *laya* means becoming absorbed, *prakṛtilayā* refers to those beings who after death, will come back and take birth into a future existence on this earth plane and become absorbed in nature.

A *yogin*, however, attaining the seedless state of *samādhi* when giving up his/her mortal existence will enjoy the pleasure and peace of contemplative absorption during the period of their divine existence. The varying worlds (*lokas*) of celestial beings are discussed more in Chapter III.

I.20 ŚRADDHĀ VĪRYA SMṚTI SAMĀDHI PRAJÑĀ PŪRVAKA ITAREṢĀM

Śraddhā *= faith*
Vīrya *= vigor, power*
Smṛti *= memory*
Samādhi *= contemplation*
Prajñā *= discernment, wisdom, insight*
Pūrvakaḥ *= precedes*
Itareṣām *= for the others*

Others (Who Follow The Path Of The Prescribed Effort) Adopt The Means Of Reverential Faith, Energy, Repeated Recollection, Concentration And Real Knowledge (And Thus Attain *Asaṃprajñāta Samādhi*).

Patañjali gives five specific steps for attaining *asaṃprajñāta samādhi*:

1) *Śraddhā* - faith
2) *Vīrya* - Energy
3) *Smṛti sādhana* - sustained memory
4) Concentration
5) Real Knowledge

> *Śraddhā coupled with vīrya is a powerful and dynamic duo that can bring the practitioner to the most expansive form of asaṃprajñāta samādhi.*

l) Tranquility and faith in this *sūtra* are known as *śraddhā,* which is a deep reverential faith that sustains us through life's difficult challenges. In this instance, it does not mean just satisfying one's own curiosity by gathering knowledge of scripture, teachings or teachers. Instead it is coupled with tranquility because it is *sattvic* in nature. It is a form of composure and serenity that is ongoing, giving us trust in the divine legions that protect and guide us within every aspect of our lives. *Śraddhā* is a powerful and necessary force, not just for the realization of the highest form of *asaṃprajñāta samādhi*, but to help us here on earth to live a more loving and grace-filled life by trusting in divine guidance.

2) *Śraddhā* and *vīrya* go together. Enthusiasm is known as *vīrya.* It is difficult to define *vīrya* in English. This word has so many layers and components. It is a formidable combination of energy, fortitude, stamina and also enthusiasm and unwavering steadiness. If there is unwavering faith (*śraddhā*) coupled with *vīrya*, it is a powerful and dynamic duo that can bring the practitioner to the most expansive form of *asaṃprajñāta samādhi* (*samādhi* without seed).

> *When the memory is purified, the mind will appear to be devoid of its own nature.*

3) The next suggested way to attain this coveted *samādhi* state is memory. Memory is known in Sanskrit as *smṛti*. It comes from *sma* meaning to remember and is known as repeated recollection. It is considered to be a principal aspect of devotional practice. *Smṛti* is one of the *vṛttis* or non-painful mind waves, but it can become painful if the *ahaṁkāra* or ego gets involved. *Smṛti* is a requisite with *śraddhā* and *vīrya* in how it can help in experiencing *asaṃprajñāta samādhi.*

There are stages of practice known as *smṛti sādhana*. When the memory is purified, the mind will appear to be devoid of its own nature. And only the object contemplated upon will remain illumined by the mind. As the mind becomes permanently established in this one-pointedness the memory becomes permanently established. The suggested object contemplated in *smṛti sādhana* (purification of the memories stored in the subconscious) would be on God or whatever object or form that God represents. Here, in this sūtra, it is suggested that the practitioner contemplate a mantra representing the vibratory sensation of God. Because the *sūtras* emphasize *Īśvara* and the sound vibration relating to *Īśvara* that dates back to the beginning of creation, it is suggested the practitioner repeat and contemplate upon the meaning of "Om" (I:27), the sound that invokes His/Her presence.

> *If when we are engaged in worldly pursuits, we can keep in mind the object of spiritual contemplation and carefully notice that it is never absent from our mind, we may be said to be working, established in a yogic state."*
>
> *-Swami Hariharānanda*

Swami Hariharānanda has stated, "Without *smṛti sādhana* pure consciousness cannot be realized. Cultivation of memory can be practiced in the midst of all actions of life, walking, sitting or lying down. If when we are engaged in worldly pursuits, we can keep in mind the object of spiritual contemplation and carefully notice that it is never absent from our mind, we may be said to be working, established in a yogic state." Another suggestion for *smṛti sādhana* is that if one practices the chant of Om (*prāṇava*), it will bring into the mind an eternally emancipated God and that memory would be fixed. Here when Swamiji says "fixed," he means memory retention of both the sound and form of that all omnipotent being.

Swami Hariharānanda 's commentaries give other suggestions on *smṛti sādhana.* "The highest practice relates to the constant remembrance of the discrimination of *puruṣa* and *prakṛti* (II:17 – II:27). This is the chief means of cleansing the mind through the form of *smṛti sādhana.*"

This form of *sādhana* is the practice of continual self-observation, watching for the slightest disturbance of fluctuations (*vṛttis*) in the field of the mind (*citta*) and stopping any fluctuations in either mind or body before they can take form. In *smṛti sādhana*, it is important to watch what is rising in the field of the mind and keep the mind undisturbed in a tranquil and neutral state.

4) By holding the mind repeatedly on a subject, memory and recollection are obtained and this leads to concentration.

5) This concentration then would lead to supreme knowledge and to *kaivalya* (liberation). As it says in Vyāsa's commentaries, "In such a mind dawns the light of discriminative knowledge by which a *yogin* understands the real nature of things."

Again, *śraddhā* and *vīrya* are so important along with memory, concentration and discernment to realize the state of *asaṃprajñāta samādhi*. Buddha said in the Dhammapada, "all sorrows can be cured through good conduct, reverential faith, enthusiasm, remembrance, concentration and correct knowledge."

I.21 TĪVRA SAMVEGĀNĀM ĀSANNAḤ

Tīvra *= keen intent*
Saṁvegānām *= with great speed*
Āsannaḥ *= sitting very close*

Those With Intense Ardor Achieve Concentration And The Result Thereof Quickly.

The word *saṁvegānām* means with great rapidity, it also means detachment (to a result) at the same time. It is an aptitude combined with a sense of reverence in devotional practice and an ardor to move towards something. Endowed with latent impressions of detachment, full of enthusiasm and energy (*vīrya*), the devotee engages him/herself with intensity in attaining the path of liberation. With this kind of intensity, the aspirant gathers divine momentum as he/she unfolds into the essence of the union of *yoga*.

As it says in Vālmīki's' Rāmāyana:

"He who is confused and has no vigor in him, alone will be depending on fate or good luck. Heroic, self-reliant men should not worship at the altar of fate. He who has the capacity to overcome the freaks of fate by his personal endeavor can never be cowered by a fate, which frustrates the hopes of men. An unvanquishable mind that knows no dejection and has great dexterity are the factors that ensure successes in any endeavor. Let not the mind slip into grief. Where valor is present, sorrow can be effectively checked. None of the ends of human life can be attained by a man who has no stamina in him."

I.22 MṚDU MADHYĀDIMĀTRATVĀT TATO'PI VIŚEṢAḤ

Mṛdu *= mild*
Madhya *= medium*
Adhimātratvat *= from full, intense*
Tataḥ *= thereupon*
Api *= also*
Viśeṣaḥ *= differentiation, distinction*

On Account Of The Methods Being Slow, Medium And Speedy (Intense), Even Among Those *Yogins* Who Have Intense Ardor, There Are Differences.

Patañjali, here describes three types of students:

1) Mild (*Mṛdu, meaning soft*)
2) Medium (*Madhya*)
3) Intense (*Adhimātratvat)*

Patañjali further divides each of these into three more parts:

1) Mildly mild, moderately mild and intensely mild
2) Mildly moderate, moderately moderate and intensely moderate
3) Mildly intense, moderately intense and intensely intense

No, we are not referring here to the different flavors of salsa! This is the varying practices as well as the varying constitutions of students. If we are one or the other, we are not stuck with this label but can change over time according to the consistency of our practice. Even if we are a mildly mild student, we can change with the aid of our practice to become mildly moderate and so forth.

Intense or speedy does not mean aggressive or goal-oriented but means with sustained ardor. This is a *sattvic* state of serenity that includes *śraddhā* or reverential faith. This is considered to be the best means of attaining *kaivalya*, or liberation, which is the ultimate essence of *yoga*.

Mr. Iyengar used to shout out in a class, "Bring me more blankets ... she's a mild student of *yoga* and needs a soft surface." At other times, he would loudly declare, "Take away his blanket, he's an intense student of *yoga* and needs a hard surface."

> *Mild....Medium....Intense.....*
> *We are not referring to different flavors of Salsa!*

1) A mild student of *yoga* is likened onto green wood; all smoke — but does not quite light and catch flame.
2) A medium student is sometimes compared to dry kindling that bursts into flame. They are enthusiastic about learning, and then after a while, the flame is not sustained but it appears to be extinguished — and then it may burst into flame once more.
3) An intense student is one who consistently sustains their faith, enthusiasm and energy. They have a natural and intuitive feeling of remembrance that lies within the depth of their psyche. Their learning comes from a "knowing" not a struggling with intellectual concepts.

> *"Take away his blanket, he's an intense student of yoga and needs a hard surface."*
>
> *- B.K.S. Iyengar*

These three methods of mild, medium and intense can be compared to the three *guṇas*. The *tamasic* student takes more effort but eventually the wood dries and can catch the flame. The *rajasic* student whose overly enthusiastic nature is up and down, is unable to sustain a state of consistency. But, as they continue with their practice, it can morph into a *sattvic* state of awareness.

The *sattvic* student is steady and consistent in taking the practice far beyond the mat into every aspect of life. They maintain a steady flame of quiet enthusiasm and faith. They usually do not flare up and then die out like the kindling. The *sattvic* student keeps burning without end like an eternal flame igniting the light in others.

> *The sattvic student just keeps burning without end like an eternal flame that ignites the light in others.*

A *sattvic* student can be seen as an intense practitioner of *yoga*. When we are in this *sattvic* state, there is seeing beyond the form of the teacher or scripture. This is known as *darshan*, from *dṛṣ*, meaning to see, to really see, to understand beyond the words or the form. The *sattvic* or serene practitioner will not so much hear the words, as they will feel the *prāṇa* or energy behind the words. The teachings reawaken something within them, a remembrance of memories stored within the hidden depths of their being.

EXERCISE:

Please Discuss or Journal on the Following Questions:

1) *Would you consider yourself a mild, medium or intense student? Why?*
2) *If you are a teacher of yoga or any other subject, have you had to adapt your teaching style according to the type of student before you? Please Explain.*

I.23 ĪŚVARAPRAṆIDHĀNĀDVĀ

Iś *- to wish*
Vara *– to fill*
Pra *– to bring forth*
Ṇi *- liking*
Dhāna *= wealth, abundance*
Vā *= or*

(Or) *Samādhi* Is Attained From Special Devotion And Dedication To *Īśvara*.

(Or) Surrender To *Īśvara*.

Īś means wish and *var* is to fill. *Pra* is to bring forth *ṇi* means liking, being drawn toward and *dhāna* means wealth. *Īśvara* would then mean to fill with wishes and bring forth the wealth.

Īśvara is not external. It is the internal core of being. *Īśvara* is the inner *guru* and companion of the soul. It is the *parabrahma*, *paramātman* and *parapuruṣa*. In the Vedas, *Īśvara* is depicted as the friend and the teacher of the most ancients. The teacher of teachers, *Īśvara* is so expansive that there is no equal. It is a special *puruṣa* that has no karmic bondage in the past nor will have any in the future. Even liberated beings have had a previous state of bondage, but *Īśvara* is beyond that, being always free, liberated and supreme.

Īśvara is a particular being whose power, knowledge and consciousness are so excessive that there is no parallel. This being is freed from all latent impressions and nescience beyond the understanding of an ordinary being.

> *To practice Īśvara praṇidhāna, we would develop a longing for that universal consciousness. Our desire to return to the source would become so strong that all we can think about is the beloved (Īśvara). Whatever we think about is what we manifest. And so the more we think about our divine source the closer we come to that universal communion.*

In surrendering to *Īśvara*, it is not done with the ego as the doer; it is a devotional dedication and offering to God of the actions in all of life done through our mind, our words and our deeds. It is said that when a devotee surrenders to *Īśvara*, that the energy field we call *Īśvara* moves towards them and favors them with grace and

fulfillment of their wishes. From this grace, the aspirant obtains *samādhi* and the state of liberation (*kaivalya*). It is through *Īśvara praṇidhāna* that one can reach *asaṃprajñāta* or the most expanded state of *samādhi* as explained in I:17.
There are different degrees to the way in which we can open our hearts to *Īśvara.* Some people are hardened and embittered through hardships. When life's challenges seem insurmountable they feel crushed beneath life's burdens. Life is so overwhelming to them that they cannot even offer a prayer or think about anything else but their problems. In facing adversities, others grow stronger and welcome life's difficulties as God's gift, in order to expand their awareness and learn greater compassion for others.

Some feel closer to the creator through hardships while others feel increasingly disconnected and abandoned. They may become hardened and embittered, sometimes depressed, feeling betrayed, even cursing "God." They struggle internally and externally, unable to relinquish their grip on the way things have always been or the way they think it should be. This inflexibility and unwillingness to change can cause a great deal of emotional as well as physical pain and turmoil. As we know in *yoga*, pain comes not so much from our changing situations but from our attachments to keeping the status quo.

Life's challenges and hurdles can cause some people to deepen their faith in a higher power, while others may buckle under the weight of life's challenges feeling alone and abandoned by their God or former beliefs.

In the *Yoga Sūtras*, you will find that Patañjali does not mention and delineate the varying paths of *yoga*. He never separated the human being into categories of physical (*haṭha*), mental (*rāja*), emotional (*bhakti*), intellectual (*gñāna/jñāna*) and vital (*tantra* and *karma).* However, it is possible to trace and correlate various verses in the *sūtras* with the corresponding paths known as *mārgas* or "Paths of *Yoga*."

This *sūtra* is the basis for *bhakti yoga*, which is the path where we transform emotion into devotion for the Divine. It is the opening of the subtle heart and to feel the ecstasy of Divine fulfillment. In *bhakti,* there are several different moods that we come to God with in offering ourselves to the Divine. One mood could be as the child to the parent or the parent to the child. For example, *Bāla* (baby) Kṛṣṇa, is a form of the Divine some women worship as their child. Others may worship God as a friend or as the lover to the beloved like the *bhakti* saint Mirabai in the 15th century India who loved Kṛṣṇa. She wandered the streets drunk with the love of Kṛṣṇa, singing poetry and dancing for her beloved. This is reminiscent of the Catholic Church,

> *Bhakti yoga is the path where we transform emotion into devotion for the Divine. It is the opening of the subtle heart and feeling the ecstasy of Divine fulfillment.*

where a nun is considered to be the bride of Jesus. There are stories of those who relate to God as the enemy, they may curse and be angry with God. *Yogis* say even in cursing God, it is a wonderful thing because it means that God is never far from our mind. Whatever we think about is what we manifest. And so the more we think about our Divine Source the closer we come to that Universal Communion. It is said in *bhakti* that when we take one step toward the Divine, it takes one thousand steps toward us.

To practice this *sūtra*, *Īśvara*, can be seen as the beloved and we, the individual, as the lover. In *bhakti*, the lover moves toward the beloved but does not consummate the union. Instead, the lover maintains a state of separation so that he/she can worship and honor the Divine. Throughout the ages, great artists, writers, poets and musicians sometimes maintained distance from the object of their love in order to fan the flames of their creativity.

In the practice of Īśvara praṇidhāna the realization dawns that the Universal is already within us. When we have devotion to that essence we do not have to leave this world but can stay within this world and live a life of dedication and devotion in true joy and bliss.

To practice *Īśvara praṇidhāna*, we would develop a longing for that universal consciousness. Our desire to return to the Source would become so strong that all we can think about is the beloved (*Īśvara*). That beloved may take a form of a religious figure, or anything inspirational or it can be a feeling, a vibrational sensation of longing for something other than this world. Some people have described this as "wanting to go home."

Each time we shed the tears of longing for our Creator, the heart opens a little bit more. In maintaining the separation from the beloved, we can honor and worship the Divine from afar without merging into it. Eventually, our desire becomes so great that we finally offer our entire being and become One with that Universal presence. If we were to follow Patañjali's suggestion in this *sūtra*, of devotion to *Īśvara* the state of *samādhi* WOULD be emminent.

Both *bhakti* and *gñāna yoga* is illustrated in the story of the moth and the nightingale. A moth fluttered into a garden on a beautiful summer's night when the sky was the color of a sheaf of the blue lotus, and the scent of night-blooming jasmine wafted through the air. The moth was drawn by a melodious sound. As he followed it, he found a nightingale weeping with tears streaming down her little face. The moth said, "Nightingale, what is wrong?" The nightingale tearfully replied, "Can you not see? I am serenading my beloved, the rose." As she spoke, the tears of joy were streaming from the outer corners of her eyes, and the tears of sorrow were descending from the inner corners.

The nightingale is a symbol of *bhakti* yoga. She was simultaneously experiencing the agony and the ecstasy in maintaining the separation so she could worship her beloved, the rose. The moth thought about this for a moment and said, "Come nightingale, let me show you what true love is." The moth found a lamp's flame in the garden. He spiraled around it and then dove into its center and was consumed by the flame, becoming one with it.

The moth represents the path of *gñāna* where we use our intellect to transcend the intellect. The moth consumed itself in the light of the flame of the Divine becoming one with *Īśvara*. The nightingale went on serenading the rose while shedding tears of agony and ecstasy in her separation from God.

This wonderful story demonstrates the difference between the *bhakti yogi* and the *gñāna yogi*. Special devotion to *Īśvara* can be both the *bhakti* of the nightingale or *gñāna*, the moth. One would be the worship and longing for the Divine and the other would be merging into and becoming one with the Divine.

The approach of the *gñāna* is more of an intellectual approach. It uses discrimination, dedication, detachment as well as devotion in the realization of *Īśvara.* In this approach, we use our mind and our intellect, to continually remember, 'we are One…we are One…we are One' until finally, like the moth to the flame, we dissolve into the sea of Oneness, or the blissful ocean of light. A *gñāni yogi* is like the sugar man, who walks into the ocean with his ruler to measure its depth and in the process dissolves into the sea and becomes one with it.

In bhakti, it is as if we are the lover and Īśvara is the beloved. We feel the agony of separation from our beloved Source and cry tears of joy that we can love so much and tears of sorrow that we are still separated from our Source.

In *bhakti yoga*, we can simply offer to our beloved, which can take the form of family, children, or the objects of our affection. We offer, as the Bhagavad Gītā says, the Inbreath to the Outbreath and to all of nature that touches our lives daily. We can offer ourselves to our work and to menial tasks such as washing dishes where the kitchen becomes our temple and the sink our altar. The 15th century monk, Brother Lawrence said that he felt closer to God in the scullery doing dishes with the love of God than he did in the prayer pews.

As the well-known poet, Khalil Gibran says in his beautiful work, *The Prophet*, "Work is Love made visible. And if you cannot work with love but only with distaste, it is better that you should leave your work and sit at the gate of the temple and take alms of those who work with joy." He also said, "You work that you may keep pace with the earth and the soul of the earth."

The story of the moth and the nightingale brings up the question, what is greater, *bhakti* or *gñāna*. Which is the best approach to realizing *Īśvara* and in turn *samādhi*. The ancients believed it is best to follow the grain of our nature. In *gñāna yoga* there is a phrase of '*Neti Neti*,' truth is not this, not that. In *bhakti yoga*, we would say '*iti, iti*' truth *is* this, it *is* that. *Bhakti* is life affirming. Through *bhakti*, which this *sūtra* represents, we come to find God in everything from the tiniest insect to the loftiest sage.

It is interesting to note that throughout the Yoga Sūtras, Patañjali never mentions the word love. In this *sūtra*, he mentions "through special devotion" to *Īśvara* the state of *samādhi* is imminent. *Īśvara* has many definitions throughout the *sūtras* but is never defined as love.

WHAT IS THIS THING CALLED LOVE?

> *It is interesting when we say, "fall in love."*
>
> *I don't know why we don't say, "rise in love."*

Perhaps what we call love, is not something that we have to strive to cultivate. Instead it is interesting to think of love as something already inherent within us. Like in the practices of *yoga*, when we remove the debris that we have accumulated in our life the Divine reveals itself. There is nowhere to go but only to let go into the realization that we are already one with the Eternal.

Love is like that. It is an inherent state. It's already there. If we can only remove the impediments that cover its light, so it can shine through. We don't have to try to love more or feel guilty when we can't forgive an injustice. When the core of our heart feels this thing called love, the sensation will pour out of us and others will feel it as unconditional love. In true unconditional love, we can love someone without expecting love in return. They feel safe in our presence because they know instinctively that we can see the divine essence within them.

It is interesting when we say, "fall in love." I don't know why we don't say, "rise in love." I think on a spiritual level, falling in love may be falling into the realm of *maya*, into the realm of illusion. In this illusory realm, we see only one intimate, special relationship, rather than holding all beings equally in our hearts. I think of this as *Īśvara praṇidhāna*. I feel that we are connecting more deeply with this great invisible and formless teacher of the most ancients who represents the ultimate in compassion.

> *"Work is Love made visible. And if you cannot work with love but only with distaste, it is better that you should leave your work and sit at the gate of the temple and take alms of those who work with joy."*
>
> *-Khalil Gibran*

> *When the core of our heart feels this thing called love, the sensation will pour out of us and others will feel it as unconditional love.*

When our heart is filled with this awareness, it's not just in our heart center that we feel this awareness, but in every cell of our being and it brings incredible closeness to this universal energy called *Īśvara*. As we feel that communion, it manifests like the rays of the sun in every direction to the atmosphere and those around us. Even if we've had problems with someone or challenges in a situation with others, we will start seeing their journey as our own. We will begin to see and feel the broken hearts of others. I often say, "Can we can meet everyone as if they have a broken heart." This can help to expand our hearts in ever increasing degrees into the growing field of compassion that is *Īśvara.*

> *Can We Meet Everyone As If They Have A Broken Heart?*

The Dalai Llama says, "love plus non-attachment equals compassion." Patañjali never mentions the word 'love' in the *yoga sūtras* but the essence of compassion is considered to be *Īśvara*. There are different degrees in which compassion evolves in the *yogin*. When we feel we've reached the finality and the intensity of feeling, there are new gateways that open that bring us into the fullness of what compassion means. This is realization of *Īśvara* and the immersion in the sea of *saṃsāra* and lifting above to hold the consciousness of that place where there is no suffering, no pain, only the bliss of oneness.

This is in the fulfillment of the *samādhi* consciousness that comes through devotion to *Īśvara* who fills and fulfills us with wishes of bliss of the Divine. In *Īśvara*, there is nothing more to want, only the realization that we hold and contain all that we've ever wanted, all that ever is. In the practice of *Īśvara praṇidhāna* the realization dawns that the Universal is already within us. When we have devotion to that essence we do not have to leave this world but can stay within this world and live a life of dedication and devotion in true joy and bliss.

EXERCISE:

Please Discuss or Journal on the Following Questions:

1) *Do you consider yourself more of a bhakti or gñāna yogi or neither? Why?*
2) *If you have a personal relationship to your view of God or Īśvara, what is the 'mood,' with which you 'approach' the Divine?*
3) *Why do you think Patañjali never mentions love in the yoga sūtras?*
4) *At some point in your life, have you experienced unconditional love? Please describe the experience.*
5) *Do you find love and joy in your work? If so, what makes it fulfilling? If not, what could change to create more joy in your worklife?*

I.24 KLEŚA KARMA VIPĀKĀŚAYAIR APARĀMṚṢṬAḤ PURUṢAVIŚEṢA ĪŚVARAḤ

Kleśa *= afflictions*
Karma *= actions*
Vipāka *= fruit of actions*
Āśayaiḥ *= storehouse of impressions left by desires*
Aparāmṛṣṭaḥ *= unaffected by*
Puruṣa *= self, soul*
Viśeṣaḥ *= distinction*
Īśvaraḥ *= supreme God*

Īśvara Is a Particular Puruṣa Unaffected by Affliction, Deed, Result of Action, or The Latent Impressions Thereof.

I find the most clarifying explanation of this *sūtra* is in the commentaries of Swami Hariharānanda Āraṇya. He speaks of *kleśas*, or afflictions, as positive or negative actions and deeds that are the result of subliminal impressions. These deep impressions are due to past actions. Because they are still subsisting in the mind it is said to be due to *puruṣa.* There are many levels of *puruṣa* that eventually culminate in the most expanded form, which is *Īśvara.*

Swami Hariharānanda says, "Liberated persons are known to have had a previous state of bondage (meaning not fully liberated and free from the plane of dualities). But this is not the case for *Īśvara. Īśvara* is always *Īśvara*, omniscient and always free. The particular *puruṣa*, who on account of His eternal liberation, is unaffected even by the touch of enjoyment or suffering is called *Īśvara*."

I am paraphrasing Swamiji in his comments that say there are many *puruṣas* who have attained the state of liberation such as the *Prakṛtilayas* or other sages and saints but can slip into bondage (the earth plane) in the future. With *Īśvara*, this is not possible.

Īśvara is always free and always supreme. For this reason, *Īśvara* is omniscient and always liberated.

Patañjali never mentions the word 'love' in the Yoga Sūtras but the essence of compassion is considered to be Īśvara.

I.25 TATRA NIRATIŚAYAṂ SARVAJÑABĪJAM

Tatra *= there (in Īśvara)*
Niratiśayaṁ *= unsurpassed manifestation, above the highest*
Sarvajñā *= omniscience*
Bījam *= seed*

In Īśvara, The Seed Of Omniscience Has Reached Its Utmost Development, Which Cannot Be Exceeded.

In this *sūtra, Īśvara* has been described as a particular Being whose power and knowledge is unparalleled. There are several *sūtras* describing *Īśvara* in a variety of ways. *Īśvara* is timeless and eternal; *Īśvara* is omnipotent and omnipresent; the name of *Īśvara* is *Om*. This *sūtra* focuses on *Īśvara* as that Being where the seeds of omniscience have reached the fullest of its expanded state and cannot be exceeded. This *sūtra* relates to *Īśvara* as being omniscient. This word refers to feeling and compassion, and here *Īśvara* would relate to the most expanded state of compassion and feeling that is possible.

There seem to be different degrees as to how compassion arises. First it comes out of our feeling for others, it is usually silent and does not express itself through tears and sentimentality. It is a feeling that sometimes wants to grow bigger when our heart center thinks it can't hold anymore. When this feeling arises and begins to expand, we may even feel and hear the bone of the sternum that protects our heart center, trying to crack open. At first we may think our heart is not big enough to contain the outflowing of love that wants to spill forth. As we continue our practice there is an outpouring of love for all Beings. When there is no attachment or personality in that love, it is known as compassion. As the compassion grows, sometimes without our conscious knowledge, the heart begins to let go of its past protections and defenses. It gradually lets go of old hurts and grievances, which gives space for it to expand even more.

This process reminds me of this particular *Īśvara* that has reached the farthest spans of omniscience, feeling and compassion. In this state, it holds all creation and creatures, both sentient and insentient within the vast periphery of its Being. Its energy field is so magnificent and magnanimous that it can hold the planetary creation (and perhaps other planets) within the scope of its feeling and compassion. After all, the term *Iś* means to wish and *var* means to fill. This great Being in its omniscience fulfills all our wishes to the point where there is nothing else to want. Everything we have ever wanted is already granted. We have and hold all past present and future desires within us at this very moment. To know this is to know that Great Being called *Īśvara*.

I am so excited about this *sūtra* because it helps me to understand that there is no *ultimate* state that one can achieve in enlightenment.

This *sūtra* is a reminder that there are many degrees, and stages that one goes through to experience the fullness of any state. We unfold gradually moving from the tiny seed within us to the fullest extent of omniscience. Perhaps we cannot reach that fullest extent, but there is always a movement of expansion where our hearts are able to embrace more and more at vast distances. When we think we cannot expand our consciousness and compassion any further, we have only to breathe, let go and the space opens. This *sūtra* is a reminder to me that this thing we call "the spiritual life" never ends, that there are always new places to go and new spaces to explore that bring us to the farthest edges of the Universal awareness to find that the outer and inner are one.

I.26 SA EṢA PŪRVEṢAM API GURUḤ KĀLENĀNAVACCHEDĀT

Saḥ *= he/she*
Pūrveṣām *= of the ancients*
Api *= even*
Guruḥ *= teacher*
Kālena *= by time*
Anavacchedāt *= unconditioned, uncut, from*

***Īśvara* Is The Teacher Of Even The Most Ancients. This Teacher Of Former Teachers Is Unlimited And Unconditioned By Time (In His/Her Omnipotence).**

This *sūtra* describes the original essence of *Īśvara* saying that He/She had full powers such as omnipotence (being present everywhere). The power of *Īśvara* dates back to the beginning as well as present cycles of creation.

As the Teacher of All Teachers, even the most Ancients, *Īśvara* is the origin of all paths and lineages of *yoga* leaders and teachings. If we were to release our ego's concept of separation and follow the thread of *yoga* back far enough, we could find and experience a common point of convergence in this powerful energetic force of creation known as *Īśvara*. With this said, it seems as if it would be an illusion to see the end results of any *yoga* methodology as separate from one another. It seems as if all paths and methodologies would merge into one another when they are traced back far enough to their common ancestral roots of *Īśvara*.

Note: Īśvara manifests throughout every chapter of the sūtras, emphasizing the importance of devotion and surrender to this vast Universal Source that is the Teacher even of the most Ancients.

I.27 TASYA VĀCAKAḤ PRAṆAVAḤ

***Tasya** = of (Īśvara)*
***Vācakah** = word, expressive, signifying*
***Praṇavaḥ** = mystic sound "OM"*

The Name Of *Īśvara* Is The Mystic Symbol Of "*OM.*"

Many years ago, when attending the European Yoga Conference in Switzerland in 1983, Sir T.K.V. Desikachar took the stage. He was strong and powerful in his concern about "*Om*." He emphatically stated that it was a sacred symbol and should not be brandished about on T-shirts, in tattoos, on bags, or on clothing. He also made a startling statement that I still remember decades later. "*Prāṇava*" his voice boomed over the microphone, "is not *Om*." The word *Prāṇava* means to bring forth (*prā*) the name (*ṇava*). This *sūtra* does not say that the name of *Īśvara* is *Om*. *Prāṇava* simply means to bring forth the name. That name can be many things in many cultures. It is different in all religions. Whatever the name of God is for a devotee in any culture or religion, let them use it. It doesn't have to be *Om*."

The ancient sound *Om* also means "the word." As it is stated in the Bible, John 1:1, Genesis, "In the beginning was the word. The word was with God, and the word was God."

However, throughout the ages, many sages and *rishis* have designated the sound of *Om* as the sound principle of creation and relate it to *Īśvara,* the Absolute. This is a powerful vibratory sound that can be heard within as well as around the body.

Here in the Yoga Sūtras, *OM* is designated as the vibratory frequency of *Īśvara*, the teacher of all former teachers, unlimited by time or place. In ancient yogic texts, *OM* is considered to be the sound that gave birth to creation. *OM*, the symbol of *yoga*, also means, 'the word.' Genesis of the Bible, John 1:1 begins, "In the beginning was the word. The word was with God, and the word was God." Ancient Eastern scriptures say that the vibrational sound of *OM* gives birth to form. *OM* is the beginning and the endless vibration of the physical, subtle and causal states of being. Its vibration pervades every cell of our body and particle of our Universe. *OM* is considered the teacher of even the most ancients. It is the symbol of the eternal cosmic vibration we call God (Goddess).

Om is said to be the sound principle of the absolute, and through its vibration, brought creation into Being. The different syllables of *OM* vibrate different energy centers within the human body. *Om* is the vibration in every organ, gland and cell within our being as well as the echo of the planetary and universal sound of creation.

By listening or saying the sound *OM*, the significance of *Īśvara praṇidhāna*, or the surrender or devotion to God, naturally brings the mind to thoughts of the Universal.
My Sanskrit teacher, Dr. David Teplitz speaks about the significance of *Om*. He taught that *OM* or *AUM* is known as *Śabda-Brahman*, or the sound of God, as it is the only phonetic symbol of *Brahman*. In *OM*, all the sounds of the Sanskrit alphabet are found. It is believed that there can be no idea or thought without a corresponding name, word or sound. Sound is inseparably associated with ideation such as the idea of *Brahman* that is beyond the creator. The three syllables of *AUM* represent the holy trinity of the East, *Brahma* (the Creator), *Viṣṇu* (The Sustainer) and *Śiva* (the Destroyer or Transformer).

I.28 TAJJAPAS TADARTHA BHĀVANAM

***Tad (taj)** = that*
***Japaḥ** = repetition*
***Tad** = that (om)*
***Artha** = meaning*
***Bhāvanam** = reflection*

Repeat It (*OM*), Reflect And Contemplate Its Meaning.

When the sound of *OM* is uttered mentally or verbally, the vibratory current arises from the heart and moves into the brain through the *vijñāna nāḍī* (the subtle energy current that connects the heart center with the brain). This vibration awakens the expansive *sahasrāra*, in the crown *cakra*, which unites energies of the heart and brain as one. In this state, the knowledge of the cosmos and the interrelationship of the microcosm and macrocosm reveal itself. In the *Māṇḍūkya Upaniṣad*, the method has been poetically described: "*Brahman* or the God within the heart, is the target, the mystic syllable of *OM* is the bow and the self or ego is the arrow."

The ancient *rishis* who were the seers and the scribes that have preserved these teachings, have written that there is no other word or sound that can bring about calmness of mind as the sound of *OM*. This mystic syllable is to be repeated with contemplation and devotion and through such chanting, the supreme soul is revealed.

OM AND THE HOLY TRINITY

These three ways in which the one Godhead manifests is known as the Holy Trinity (*Trimūrthi*) of *Brahma*, *Viṣṇu* and *Śiva* known in the west as the Father, the Son and the Holy Ghost. *AUM* is the symbol of these three forces that manifest as one.

OM is accurately chanted as *AUM*. The syllable *A* represents *Brahma*, the creator that brings forth the procreative life force. *U* (oo) is the sound principle of *Viṣṇu*, which is the energy that sustains and supports creation. The sound of *M* where the lips are closed represents *Śiva*, the energy field that destroys and dissolves in order to transform. This sound releases old forms and pre-existing patterns for the new to be born.

When the lips are sealed, there is a fourth vibratory current, the sound of *mng*. This sound current is produced by bringing the top of the tongue (not the tip) upward to touch the roof of the mouth. This sound vibrates the cerebral plexus, and is done by opening the mouth slightly as if preparing to start chanting the next cycle of *AUM*, which is symbolic of the next cycle of creation.

Brahma, the creator, is said to reside in the first *cakra*, *mūlādhāra*, at the base of the spine. *Mūlā* means base and *dhāra* means support, *mūlādhāra* means base support. It is the element of earth and the sense of smell. *Brahma* resides with his feminine consort *Saraswatī*.

> *"Om is the bow*
> *the mind*
> *is the arrow*
> *and Brahman*
> *the Universal*
> *is the Target"*
>
> *Māṇḍūkya Upaniṣad*

What follows creation (*Brahma*) is that which maintains and stabilizes that creation, which would be the Lord *Viṣṇu* who is said to dwell in the second *cakra,* known as *Svādiṣṭhāna*, which literally means, "to establish one's own place within the eternal cosmic vibration." This *cakra* holds the element of water and the sense of taste.

Lord *Viṣṇu* is said to preside here with his consort *Lakṣmī*, the post-Vedic queen of the waterways who is known for beauty, graciousness and benevolent compassion. It is *Lakṣmī* who bestows upon her devotees, success in all endeavors, liberation of consciousness, and enjoyment of life. She arises from the milky ocean of our individual and collective subconscious with the churning of the ocean of milk, which represents the cloudy depth of the subconscious psyche.

In some mythology, it is not the celestial physician who carries the nectar of immortality in the cup of the moon, but *Lakṣmī*. As the Goddess *Lakṣmī* arises from the unseen depth of the primordial ocean, she carries a white lotus in one hand, which is symbolic of purity of heart and integrity. With the other hand, she showers gold coins upon her devotees representing spiritual and material abundance. In another hand, she holds a golden vessel of *amṛta*, the soma, nectar or fluid of immortality.

Lakṣmī and *Viṣṇu* represent the spiritual power that is in every atom, cell and molecule of our Being. It is the energy that pulses through the procreative centers of all species. It is the *prāṇa* of our breath, the beat and rhythm of our heart. The word *Viṣṇu* means all pervasive. It is the all-pervading *prāṇa* or life force that maintains our body as well as the substratum of the Universe.

Śiva is said to reside in the *sahasrāra cakra*, the thousand-petaled lotus at the crown of the head. *Śiva* is a hermit who was known to meditate upon Mount *Kailāsaḥ*, his Himalayan abode that represents the crown pole of our being. *Śiva* is usually called the "Destroyer" but he is the energy that dissolves the old for the new to come forth. *Śiva* represents the dissolution of old structures that no longer serve. He represents change. *Śiva* is both the ashes and the phoenix that rises out of the ashes.

It is said that *Viṣṇu* holds the balance between *Brahma*, the creator at the base of the spine and *Śiva*, the destroyer or transformer of the energy that dwells in the crown pole of the head. *Viṣṇu* represents balanced living and like his later incarnation of *Kṛṣṇa*, symbolizes the cosmic *Līlā*, a Sanskrit word that means the "Divine play of life."

AUM is an endless vibration of the physical, subtle and causal states of consciousness. The vibration pervades every cell of our being and particle of our universe. When we chant this sound it creates a holographic resonance from the microorganisms of the body to the macrocosm of the Universe. It helps the organs to remember their normal healthy frequency and clears the channels for the dawning light of universal consciousness.

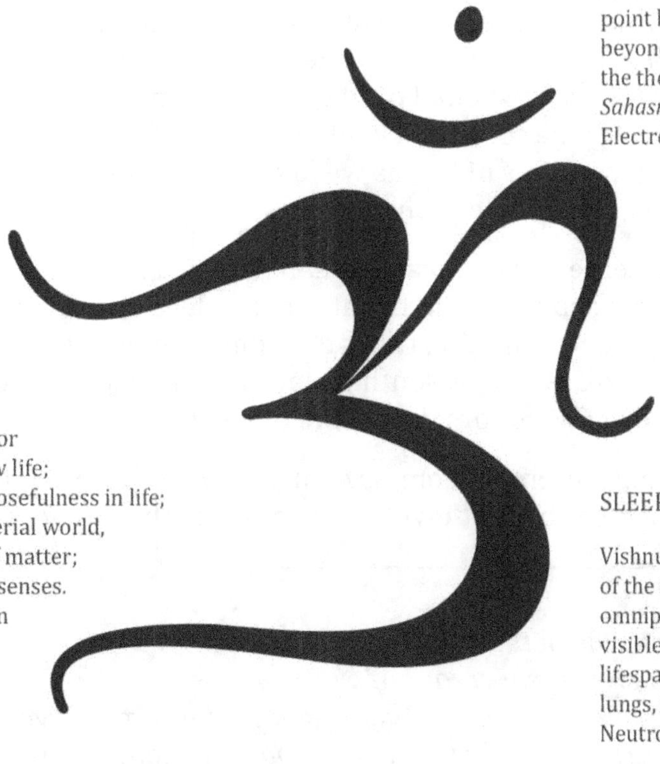

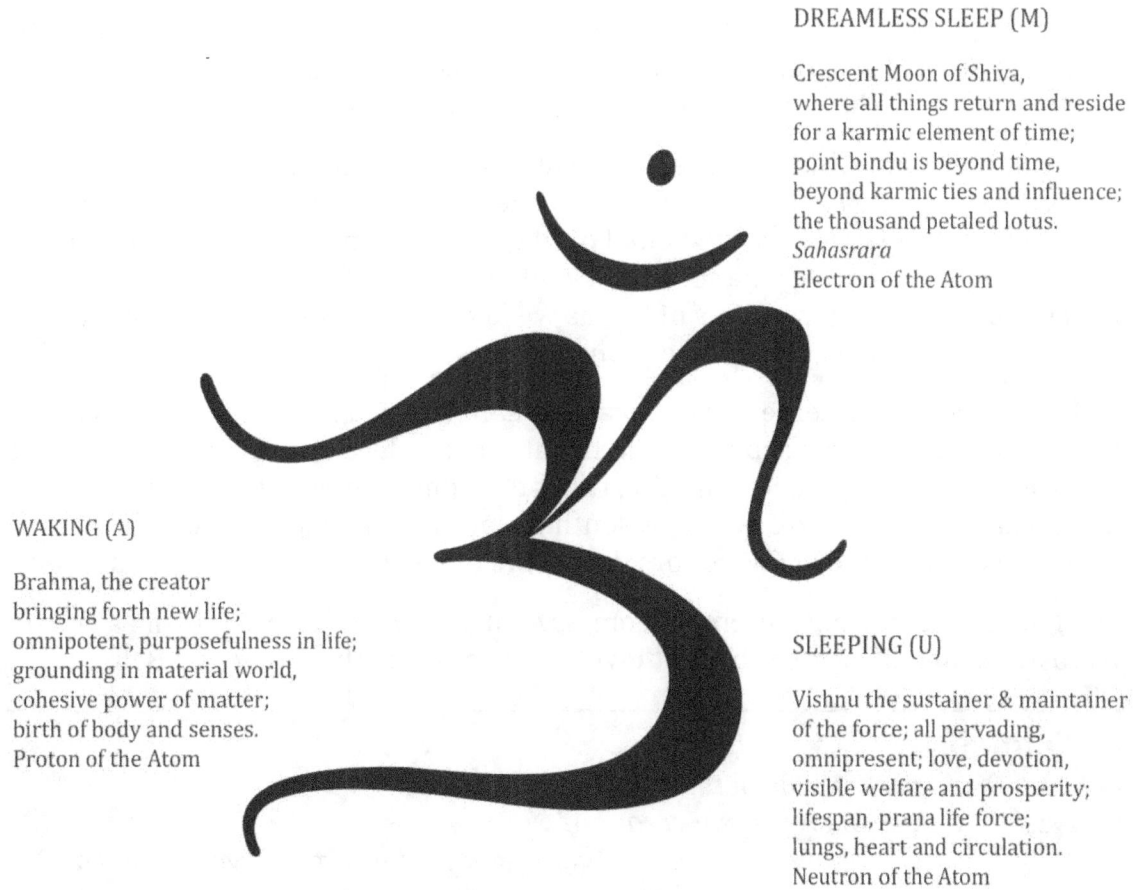

DREAMLESS SLEEP (M)

Crescent Moon of Shiva,
where all things return and reside
for a karmic element of time;
point bindu is beyond time,
beyond karmic ties and influence;
the thousand petaled lotus.
Sahasrara
Electron of the Atom

WAKING (A)

Brahma, the creator
bringing forth new life;
omnipotent, purposefulness in life;
grounding in material world,
cohesive power of matter;
birth of body and senses.
Proton of the Atom

SLEEPING (U)

Vishnu the sustainer & maintainer
of the force; all pervading,
omnipresent; love, devotion,
visible welfare and prosperity;
lifespan, prana life force;
lungs, heart and circulation.
Neutron of the Atom

OM AND THE THREE GUṆAS

OM relates to the atomic correlates of the three *guṇas*; *Guṇḍ* means to bind and the *guṇas* are the binding forces of all matter. They are active in the world around and within us. They manifest from the foods we eat to the atomic particles that comprise creation.

> ***Review of the 3 Gunas:***
> ***Sattva*** *is the principle of equilibrium, contentment, peace, harmony, and purity. It is the original state of the mind. This state of mind is ideal for spiritual practice.*
>
> ***Rajas*** *is the principle of movement and energy. It is associated with activity, restlessness, agitation, desire, aggression, will and self-seeking action. It has an outward motion.*
>
> ***Tamas*** *is the principle of inertia. It is associated with matter, density, dullness, obstruction, heaviness and darkness. It has an inward and downward motion.*
>
> *For more on the 3 Gunas, see* *guṇas* in *Samkhya Philosophy* page VIII

Brahma is the *rajas guṇa*, active in bringing forth creation. It is symbolized by the first syllable of *A* which represents the beginning and fullness of creation. It is known as the waking state or dawn of consciousness.

Viṣṇu, the *sattva guṇa*, is a state of repose, not of doing, but an aspect of "being." It is the *U* (oo) of *OM*. *Viṣṇu* represents the resting or sleeping state of awareness that lies dormant in the light of consciousness of its own dreams.

Śiva, is *tamas guṇa*, which transcends the dream into the dreamless state of sleep. *Śiva* is the sound of *M* and is symbolized by the crescent moon and the dot above in the symbol of *OM* (see chart on symbol of OM). The dot, in Sanskrit is called the *anusvāra*, which dissolves the sound back into itself. *Śiva* is *tamasic* at its very highest form, drawing the forms of life, as we know it back into the nuclear center of its own creation, to begin the cycle again.

Brahma is the proton center that activates creation. *Viṣṇu* is the neutron force that holds the proton and electron force. In the atom, the electrons that vibrate around the proton and neutron over a million times a second, can be seen as creation itself like the dance of *Śiva* and *Śakti* representing matter as we experience it through the five senses. The sound of *OM* honors the Divine essence in all of its manifestations.

OM is omnipotent, omnipresent and omniscient, known as *Īśvara*. It is the all-pervasive sound of all creation that invokes the grace of this Universal Being.

> ***EXERCISE:***
> *Please Discuss or Journal on the Following Questions:*
> 1) *How does OM represent creation?*
> 2) *What are your views on the power of sound vibration? Have you had a healing or harmful experience with sound vibration? Please Describe.*

I.29 TATAḤ PRATYAK CETANĀDHIGAMO 'PYANTARĀYABHĀVAŚ CA

***Tataḥ** = from this*
***Pratyak** = inner*
***Cetana** = Self*
***Adhigamo** = knowledge*
***Api** = also*
***Antarāya** = obstacles*
***Abhāvaḥ** = disappear*
***Ca** = and*

From This Practice All Obstacles Disappear, And Simultaneously Dawns Knowledge Of The Inner Self.

This *sūtra* refers to the practice in the previous *sūtra* of repeating and contemplating "The Word" the scriptures translate as *OM*, which is *Īśvara*. Patañjali here says something to the effect of, "from the practice of chanting *Om*, all obstacles disappear and from that dawns knowledge of the Inner Self."

With devotion to *Īśvara,* obstacles such as sickness, incompetence, doubt, and delusion disappear bringing about freedom from afflictions like nescience (*avidyā*) and other *kleśas* (II:3) which are the reasons for life's emotional pain and suffering. This *sūtra* is the extension of *Īśvara praṇidhāna* where Swami Hariharānanda refers to the revelation of the Inner Self that leads to a blissful experience of unencumbered freedom from cycles of birth, span of life and death.

Patañjali uses the word *pratyak* in this *sūtra* to refer to everything underlying *puruṣa*. He says that the word *pratyak* also refers to the word "ancient" as in the "Ancient Being of *Īśvara*." *Pratyak* then is considered to be a form of *Īśvara*. In this *sūtra*, however, *pratyak cetana* is considered to mean "One's Own Self." I define this *sūtra* as "Through devotion to *Īśvara*, knowledge dawns of the Inner Self."

> *Īśvara can either have a concept or a form or it may be formless. When it is formless, it can manifest as a sensation of fullness in every cell of our body or a feeling of being complete within every fiber of our Being.*

Note: Patañjali gives the obstacles of this realization in the following sūtra.

I.30 VYĀDHI STYĀNA SAṂŚAYA PRAMĀDĀLASYĀVIRATI BHRĀNTIDARŚANĀLABDHABHŪMIKATVĀNAVASTHITAT-VĀNI CITTAVIKṢEPĀSTE'NTARĀYĀḤ

Vyādhi = *disease*
Styāna = *dullness*
Saṃśaya = *doubt*
Pramāda = *carelessness*
Ālasya = *laziness*
Avirati = *sensuality, intemperance*
Bhrānti = *false*
Darśana = *perception*
Alabdhabhūmikatva = *failure to reach firm ground*
Anavasthitatva = *slipping down from the ground gained*
Ani = *an ending to the nine words indicating them as a group*
Citta = *mind stuff*
Vikṣepaḥ = *distraction*
Te = *these*
Antarāyāḥ = *obstacles*

Disease, Dullness, Doubt, Carelessness, Laziness, Sensuality, False Perception, Failure To Reach Firm Ground And Slipping From The Ground Gained – These Distractions Of The Mind Stuff Are The Obstacles. (Swami Satchidānanda)

What are these impediments that disturb the calm of the mind? What are they called and how many are there? There are nine obstacles that cause distraction of the mind. Swami Hariharānanda 's translation uses slightly different words:

1) **Sickness**
2) **Incompetence**
3) **Doubt**
4) **Delusion**
5) **Sloth**
6) **Non-Abstention**
7) **Erroneous Conception**
8) **Non-Attainment of Any Yogic Stage**
9) **Instability to Stay In A Yogic State**

These distractions of the mind are the impediments.

1) Illness comes from an imbalance of the *prāṇas*, the *doshas* (three bodily elements that make up the constitution) and secretions such as the endocrine system. In *yoga*, it is believed that imbalances in the *prāṇic*, or subtle body, can sift down into the cellular structure of the physical body creating what we call sickness or disease. Disease is a major obstacle of *Yogaś Citta Vṛtti Nirodhaḥ*. When the body ails, it is difficult to maintain practices of *yoga* and concentration. This is why health of the body is so important to a *yogin*.

2) Incompetence. When the mind is restless and cannot be engaged in devotional work like contemplation, it is considered incompetence or incapacity of the mind. Incompetence or listlessness is said to be due to the inability of the mind to be steady. It roams about uncontrollably.

3) Doubt can also be a form of confusion where the mind wavers from one polarity to the other such as: "perhaps it is this...or perhaps it is that." Doubt can also come from a lack of faith in a power greater than oneself. If there is doubt, *vīrya* is not possible. Without the firmness, steadfastness, enthusiasm, and faith of *vīrya* one cannot quiet the mind. To relinquish doubt, Swami Hariharānanda Āraṇya suggests in his commentary that an aspirant "must listen to instructions and contemplate them by being in the company of a calm and sure-minded preceptor."

4) Delusion – Being engaged in worldly affairs and forgetting the true nature of Self is considered to be delusion. Delusion can be countered by the continual remembrance that though we are in this world, we are not of this world.

5) Sloth – Disinclination to engage oneself in devotional practice due to dullness of body and mind is sloth. Moderation in diet, wakefulness, and enthusiasm can conquer sloth.

6) Non-Abstention stems out of the desire or thirst for or addictions to worldly objects or experiences. This can be countered through *brahmacarya* as we see in II:38, where addictions are transcended through sensual regulation.

7) Erroneous Conception is false knowledge, i.e. mistaking one thing for another. Not knowing what is to be given up or removed in our life or not knowing the means to accomplish it. In the beginning of this chapter, Patañjali speaks of incorrect perception (*viparyaya*), which is the second non-painful mind wave. In chapter II he refers to the second *kleśa* or painful mind wave as *asmitā* that is also erroneous conception but on a more universal level.

Swami Hariharānanda comments,
"Through profound devotion to God as well as to a preceptor, and study of sacred scripture false perception is removed."

8) Non-attainment of any *yogic* stage of concentration. This is due to not being fully established in any of the *yogic* states. To get established in a stage, realization of *yoga* principles is necessary.

9) Inability to stay in a *yogic* state relates to the failure to maintain the attained state (of concentration). When concentration is established, the mind-stuff (*citta*) remains firm in that attained state (*Yogaś Citta Vṛtti Nirodhaḥ*).

Note: These above mentioned obstacles are known as the foes of Yoga. " Through Īśvara praṇidhāna the impediments mentioned above disappear, because whatever are antidotes to such obstacles are obtained through special devotion to God whereby pure sattvika intellect is developed and the yogin gradually gains power with which [one] is able to resist such obstacles," writes Swami Hariharānanda Āraṇya.

These obstacles may seem insurmountable, but the previous *sūtra* says that these obstacles can be overcome through the practice of *Īśvara praṇidhāna*, which is devotion and surrender to the omnipotent, omniscience and omnipresent Self. This *Īśvara* can either have a concept or a form or it may be formless. When it is formless, it can manifest as a sensation of fullness in every cell of our body or a feeling of being complete within every fiber of our Being. When the realization of "Oneness" occurs, there is nothing more to do, to want, or to become. All Is. All obstacles and impediments can automatically drop away in this "realized state."

Note: Patañjali identifies the obstacles and gives many other ways to overcome these obstacles to Self and Universal Realization in succeeding sūtras and chapters.

I.31 DUḤKHA DAURMANASYĀṄGAMEJAYATVA ŚVĀSA PRAŚVĀSĀ VIKṢEPA SAHABHUVAḤ

Duḥka = *sorrow*
Daurmanasya = *despair or dejection*
Aṅgam = *the body*
Ejayatva = *trembling of*
Śvāsa = *disturbed inhalation*
Praśvāsā = *disturbed exhalation*
Vikṣepa = *distraction of mind, inability to concentrate*
Saha = *accompany*
Bhuvaḥ = *arising, existing*

Sorrow, Dejection, Restlessness Or Shakiness Of The Body, Inhalation And Exhalation Arise From (Previous) Distractions.

A. Sorrow is of three kinds:

1) *Ādhyātmika* – that which arises within ourselves
2) *Ādhibhautika* – inflicted by someone or something else
3) *Ādhidaivika* – through natural calamity

B. Dejection is said to be caused by unfilled desires or expectations. When we wish for something and it does not happen it can result in futility or dejection.

C. Restlessness of the body where a shock, illness or distress that upsets the body's equilibrium and puts strain on the nervous system. This can result in shakiness of the body.

D. Inhalation and exhalation reveal the irregularity and shallowness of unconscious breathing that are signs of a distracted mind. When the breath cannot be consciously controlled it can result even in "anxiety attacks." However, through the practices of *prāṇāyāma*, and conscious, volitional breathing, we can have voluntary control over our breath, strengthen our nervous system and in turn, develop a concentrated mind. *(See Chapter II, VV. 49-53 on prāṇāyāma.)*

Through the practices of prāṇāyāma, and conscious, volitional breathing, we can have voluntary control over our breath, strengthen our nervous system and in turn, develop a concentrated mind.

I.32 TAT PRATIṢEDHĀRTHAMEKATATTVĀBHYĀSAḤ

Tat *= their*
Pratiṣedha *= prevention*
Artham *= for the sake of*
Eka *= one, single*
Tattva *= subject, true principle, reality*
Abhyāsa *= checking the downward pull or continual practice*

The (Foregoing) Obstacles Can Be Prevented Or Reversed By The Continual Practice Of Concentration On One Single Principle, Or On One Subject.

Some commentaries refer to *Īśvara* as that single principle for concentration. Others say it refers to some gross principle, while yet others say that it refers to a specifically selected principle. This *sūtra* does not seem to give specifics of an object of contemplation but refers to the quality of contemplation.

To explain this *sūtra*, Swami Satchidānanda, in his commentaries, speaks of the old *yogic* adage, "Dig a well in only one place." This emphasizes the need to focus on one object or one principle. The Swami Hariharānanda commentaries say, "For practice of one principle, *Īśvara* and I-sense are the best. 'I am the observer of all the modifications that are taking place every moment in the mind' — a recollection of such as 'I' as a support of contemplation is very soothing to the mind. This is what the Upanishads call the contemplation on I-sense."

> *"Dig a well in only one place."*
> *- Yogic Adage*

EXERCISE:
Please Discuss or Journal on the Following Questions:

1) *Of the 9 Obstacles Patañjali mentions, which are you challenged by? Which do you feel are easy to overcome?*
2) *How do you overcome obstacles? Does it bear any resemblance to sūtra I.32? Please Explain.*

HOMEPLAY: *For the next week, choose one of the 9 obstacles and seek to overcome it each day using sutra I.32. Keep notes of your experiences in your sūtra diary.*

I.33 MAITRĪ KARUṆĀ MUDITOPEKṢĀṆĀṂ SUKHA DUḤKHA PUṆYĀPUṆYA VIṢAYĀṆĀṂ BHĀVANĀTAŚ CITTA PRASĀDANAM

Maitrī *= friendliness*
Karuṇā *= compassion*
Mudita *= delight*
Upekṣa *= disregard (anam = of these four)*
Sukha *= happy*
Duḥkha *= unhappy*
Puṇya *= virtuous*
Apuṇya *= wicked*
Viṣaya *= in the domain (anam = of the four)*
Bhāvanatah *= cultivating the attitudes*
Citta *= mind-stuff*
Prasādanam *= undisturbed calmness*

The Mind Becomes Purified By The Cultivation Of Feelings of Amity, Compassion, Goodwill And Indifference, Respectively Towards Happy, Miserable, Virtuous and Sinful Creatures.

This is an important sutra for creating a more grace-filled life...

The cultivation of feelings of amity, or friendliness and compassion in this instance would be extended to all who have ever crossed the path of our life. If we delight in the misfortunes of those we may see as an enemy or not our friend, our mind takes on more disturbances. However, there are instances where a person may not delight and be happy over the fortunes of their friend. There may be hidden areas of envy and even jealousy. One might pretend to be happy for them, but if things are not going well within their own life, it could be challenging to align true feelings with expressions of delight. This would reflect a mind where division and separation exists.

This *sūtra* would also apply to one we may not call friend, and even see as an "enemy." If our enemy experiences misfortune and we delight in their suffering on a subconscious level we can create more turbulence rather than serenity of mind. Purification of the mind refers to that which does not disturb the *vṛttis*, or mind waves, either on a conscious or subconscious level.

This *sūtra* is a powerful reminder to equally delight in the happiness and good fortune of friend or enemy. It is a blessed reminder to feel compassion equally for all, those who are closest to us in our life and to those who are at a distance whether across the street or across the world. This *sūtra* asks the aspirant to hold the same compassionate attitude as we would toward the misfortunes of a friend or enemy alike. In this practice, even the concept of "friend" or "enemy" dissolves into the sea of "Oneness," where the mind is no longer in division or separation.

> *Every saint has had a past, every sinner has a future.*
>
> *Kirpal Singh*

The part in this *sūtra* that says, "Indifference Respectively Toward Happy, Miserable, Virtuous and Sinful Creatures," was also difficult for me to understand. I never used the terms evil or sinful only the word forgetful. There are so many degrees of forgetfulness that may appear as "sinful." After years of pondering this *sūtra* regarding indifference, I realized that it probably did not mean cold indifference, but mental and emotional neutrality towards everyone whether they are happy or suffering, or considered to be virtuous or sinful.

As Swami Hariharānanda Āraṇya says in his commentaries, "To overlook the lapses in others is indifference. It is not positive thinking or denial but it is restraining the mind from dwelling on the frailties of others." This is so important considering a common theme throughout the Sūtras is that if we dwell on the defects of others, we take on those defects.

As the Swami continues in his commentaries, he writes, "Feelings of envy, cruel delight, malevolence or anger disturb the mind and prevent its attaining concentration. By cultivating the opposite feelings, the mind can be kept pleasant and happy, free from any disturbing element, then it can become one-pointed and tranquil."

I.34 PRACCHARDANAVIDHĀRAṆĀBHYĀṂ VĀ PRĀṆASYA

***Pracchardana** = exhale, expulsion*
***Vidhāraṇa** = retention*
***Abhyam** = by these two*
***Vā** = or*
***Prāṇasya** = of the breath*

By Exhaling And Restraining The Breath Also (The Mind Is Calmed).

Commentaries by Swami Hariharānanda Āraṇya are explicit in saying that "it is on the exhalation that the ego disentangles itself from the body and the feeling of Self in the core of the heart is moving on to the wordless, thoughtless state of concentrated awareness." He continues to say "this is possible only at the time of exhalation and not at the time of inhalation."

In Sanskrit, the word for ego is *ahaṁkāra* from *ahaṁ*, which means "I Am," and *kāra* is from *kri*, meaning to do or to act. Thus, *ahaṁkāra* would mean, "I Am Doing." The ego asserts itself on the inhalation and unravels and transforms itself on the exhalation. If we move into *āsana* on an exhalation, the action is performed in an egoless state. The *āsana* would then feel as it were being done *through* us rather than *from* us.

> *It is on the exhalation that the ego disentangles itself from the body and the feeling of Self in the core of the heart is moving on to the wordless, thoughtless state of concentrated awareness.*

If we practice breathing without attempting to focus the mind it does not result in calmness. If we practice without *dhyāna* (meditation) the mind instead of becoming calm becomes more disturbed. The *śāstras* say that the breath should be attuned to a conception of the void. When we exhale, we are to keep the mind vacant, releasing any thoughts with the out-breath. Exhaling in this way calms the thought waves that arise within the field of mind. If we exhale keeping the mind vacant, it is considered to be *prāṇāyāma*. When inhaling, there is no effort or labor for the breath, but it comes in naturally and effortlessly. As we merely observe this incoming breath, allowing it to quietly enter the gateways of the nostrils, the mind will remain calm and vacant. I call this creating space between thoughts. If however, we forcefully breathe in or pull the breath in from great distances beyond ourselves, the mind will become scattered and restless. In this state one thought gets superimposed upon the other and the mind is not vacant.

IN ĀSANA

If we move into *āsana* on our exhalation, we can keep the mind still and vacant as our ego relinquishes itself. As we inhale, it is a time to be still and unmoving, not giving the ego power. The inhalation is a time to rest, do nothing and gather our *prāṇic* energies before moving into a pose. If we exhale when moving into a pose, it becomes an egoless movement, an action of humility where every pose becomes an offering to the creator or to the "Higher Self." If *āsana* is practiced this way, the action will be an egoless action, and there will be the sensation that "the pose is being done through me," rather than "I Am *doing* the pose."

> *'The Pose Is Being Done Through Me,' rather than, 'I Am Doing The Pose.'*

To begin moving on the exhalation, not the inhalation, first the breath is drawn in horizontally across the back from the shoulders to the buttocks. On the exhalation, rather than collapsing, the spine elongates propelling one effortlessly into their chosen pose. In this way, the breath is like the symbol of the cross. The inhalation represents the horizontal expansion in service to humanity, and the exhalation is symbolic of our vertical ascension and connection to the Divine.

If there is a feeling of space and lightness within *āsana* and an organic retention of the exhalation (*bāhya kuṁbhaka*), it reflects a calm and tranquil mind that is free from fluctuations. This is the practice of *prāṇāyāma* in āsana.

There are three steps in the art of exhalation: 1) slow and deep exhalations, 2) keeping the body still and relaxed in *yoga* and in life, and 3) keeping the mind vacant without any thought.

If we can linger at the end of an exhalation and relax around its retention, it is a natural *bāhya kuṁbhaka*. Whenever we feel the need to inhale, before taking in the breath, if we can wait and relax around this urgency, a new space opens where our out breath moves us more deeply into a pose and into ourselves. The *śāstras* (scriptures) say, "The breath should be attuned to the conception of the void." When exhaling, the mind is to be kept vacant. Exhaling in this way calms the thought waves that arise in the field of the mind bringing the practitioner into a fusion of supra-consciousness. This state of consciousness can be seen as Saṁyama Yoga, which is the fusion of *dhāraṇā*, (concentration), *dhyāna* (meditation) and *samādhi* (Chapter III).

> *If we exhale when moving into a pose, it becomes an egoless movement, an action of humility where every pose becomes an offering to the Creator or to the "Higher Self."*

I.35 VIṢAYAVATĪ VĀ PRAVṚTTIRUTPANNĀ MANASAḤ STHITINIBANDHANĪ

***Viṣayavatī** = having an object of sense perception (sound, tangibility, form, savor and odor)*
***Vā** = or*
***Pravṛttiḥ** = refined activity, subtle sense perception*
***Utpannā** = uprising*
***Manasaḥ** = of the mind*
***Sthiti** = steadiness*
***Nibandhanī** = bind, fix upon*

The Development Of Higher Objective Perceptions Called Viṣayavatī Also Brings About Tranquility of Mind.

Patañjali's *Yoga Sūtras* continue to unfold, giving a myriad of ways in which the *yogin* can bring the mind waves into the ultimate quiescent state of *Yogaś Citta Vṛtti Nirodhaḥ*. Here, Patañjali suggests focusing on the object of sensory perceptions known as *viṣayavatī,* which in this instance is translated as "relating to objects" of the senses. This would mean to bring one to a heightened perception of awareness through the senses. The intent of this practice would be to bring about tranquility and steadiness (*sthiti*) of the mind.

How can we do this?

Viṣayavatī in this instance is translated as "relating to objects." This would mean to bring one to a heightened perception of awareness through the senses.

l) By using the object of the tip of the nose as a focal point of concentration, we can develop a heightened sense of smell. An example of this would be, smelling a delightful fragrance of a flower when none is present. When this happens it is sometimes thought that a particular fragrance relates to an invisible presence of a deity or saint. The sense of smell is related to the first *cakra*.

2) To focus on the tip of the tongue it is possible to develop super-sensuous taste. If we taste a very hot dish that may burn our tongue, if it is at the tip, we won't be able to taste foods until it heals. This is not true with other parts of the tongue. The sense of taste is related to the second *cakra*.

3) If we use the object of concentration at the root of the tongue, it is associated with the ear bringing about super-sensuous hearing. This also relates to verbal articulation. When we have thoughts, there is usually a verbal association in the mind. We form words corresponding to those thoughts. This would be a form of having a dialogue with our self. If we can relax the tongue, the inner ear opens and the mind moves toward a state of stillness. This sense relates to the fifth *cakra* (*viśuddhi*) located at the throat center.

4) If we focus on the palate, it brings about super-sensuous color because the optic nerve is situated above the palate. Colors become brighter and we develop not just sight with the outer eye, but deep insights into people and situations. This sense relates to the third *cakra* of *maṇipūra*.

5) To focus on the entire tongue (upper and lower) brings about super-sensuous touch. This is a heightened sense of "feeling" and an all-pervasive "touch." When this sense becomes amplified, it can embrace all of humanity. This sense relates to compassion and the fourth *cakra* of *anāhata* that lies in the subtle center of the heart.

> *As Gene Wilder Says in the movie, Little Prince ...*
>
> *"It's only with the heart that one can see clearly, what's essential is invisible to the eye."*

Vyasa gives other suggestions in this *sūtra* in which the aspirant can unravel and stabilize the turbulent modifications of the mind. He suggests using perceptions such as "the sun, the moon, the planets, jewels or lamps," and calls them "objective perceptions." The awakening of these higher perceptions, he says, "firmly stabilizes the mind, removes doubts and forms the gateway to knowledge that comes through concentration."

This heightened awareness of the five super-sensuous states can lead to faith, energy, remembrance and concentration. These suggested states of concentration can also lead to an ever-expanding sense of tranquility and a revelatory experience of the highest *puruṣa* that is *Īśvara*. One aspect of *Īśvara* is un-ending and all pervasive "touch" where one can embrace all of humanity in the ever-widening arms of universal compassion.

> *The awakening of these higher perceptions, Vyasa says, "firmly stabilizes the mind, removes doubts and forms the gateway to knowledge that comes through concentration."*

I.36 VIŚOKĀ VĀ JYOTIṢMATĪ

***Viśokā** = blissful (sorrow-less)*
***Vā** = or*
***Jyotiṣmatī** = the internal supreme light*

Or By Perception Which Is Free From Sorrow And Is Radiant, Stability of Mind Can Also Be Produced.

Jyoti means light and *Mati* relates to the mother, the divine essence of creation...

Jyotiṣmatī is the light where other greater lights are lit.

Jyoti means light and *matī* relates to the mother, the divine essence of creation. *Jyotiṣmatī* is the light where other greater lights are lit.

It is so interesting to observe how Patañjali keeps giving the *yoga* aspirant a variety of ways in which to realize the state of *samādhi.* The following commentaries of Vyasa give specific ways in which a *yoga* aspirant can bring the mind to a point of tranquility or stillness.

Imagine the Lotus in the Core of the Heart Known As the abode of Brahman. This is the Presence of a Limitless, Uninterrupted Expanse of Sky, Effulgent Like the Sky on a Cloudless Day.

Sage Vyasa

"Contemplation practiced on the innermost core of the heart brings about the knowledge of *buddhi*. That *buddhi* is resplendent like the *ākāśa*, the boundless void. *Buddhi* is perceived here as resembling the effulgent sun, moon, planet, or as a luminous jewel. When the mind is engrossed in this I-sense, it appears like a wave-less ocean, placid and limitless." These wonderful commentaries by Vyasa continue on this *sūtra*: "Reaching contemplation of *bodhisattva*, the pure 'I-sense' is the first to imagine the lotus in the core of the heart known as the abode of *brahman*. This is the presence of a limitless, uninterrupted expanse of sky, effulgent like the sky on a cloudless day. The effulgence in the heart remains objectively present in the contemplation of the pure I-sense.

"The mind engrossed in the thought of pure I-sense, appears like a waveless ocean, placid and limitless, which is pure I-sense all over. It has been said in this connection: 'By the reflective meditation on the self or self in its pure atomic form, there arises the pure knowledge of 'I am'.' This higher perception named *viśokā* is two-fold, one relating to objects, the other relating to pure I-sense. (Together) these are called *jyotiṣmatī* (effulgent) and through them, the mind of the *yogin* attains stability (and tranquility)."

> *"Brahma reveals himself in yoga to one who first contemplates on an effulgence like that of a mist, smoke, sun, air, firefly, lightening, crystal or the moon."*
>
> *Upanishads*

Swami Hariharānanda in his commentaries on Vyasa's commentaries gives specific suggestions for accessing the effulgent light. "Imagine in your heart, a limitless sky or transparent effulgence. Then think that the 'I-sense' or Self is within—'I am spread all over'—and become one with it.

Such thought brings ineffable bliss. The transparent radiant sense of ego radiating from the heart into infinity is known as *viśokā jyotiṣmatī* or effulgent light free from sorrow." *Yogins* focus this inner light emanating from the heart on an object that one wants to know. In the Upanishads it says, "Brahma reveals himself in yoga to one who first contemplates on an effulgence like that of a mist, smoke, sun, air, firefly, lightening, crystal or the moon."

These specific practices can be done at any time. They can be practiced in *āsana* and *prāṇāyāma* as well as interacting with others. This practice can continue throughout each day, even in our dreams. They can be remembered when sitting in a pose of contemplation, or cooking a meal. The light is already within us. Wherever we turn our attention, there it will be.

> *The transparent radiant sense of ego radiating from the heart into infinity is known as viśokā jyotiṣmatī or effulgent light free from sorrow*

This is such a beautiful *sūtra* because it refers to that "lamplike thing" in the heart known as *jyotiṣmatī*. *Jyoti* means light and *matī* relates to the mother, the divine essence of creation. *Jyoti* is not considered to be a big light. It is a small light and yet, a flame that never dies. It is known as the eternal flame. Even though this light in itself is not a huge flame it is steady and unwavering, where even the strongest wind cannot extinguish its light. It is the light from which other greater lights are lit. Some of those lights may become huge for a time, then eventually die out. The light of the *jyotiṣmatī* keeps on burning. There may be times in our life when that lamp or light within our heart may flicker and even seem to die out. However, even though we are not always able to perceive it, *jyotiṣmatī* is eternally present in the subtlest core of our heart.

> *Jyotiṣmatī keeps on burning. There may be times in our life when that lamp or light within our heart may flicker and even seem to die out. However, even though we are not always able to perceive it, jyotiṣmatī is always ever present in the subtlest core of our heart.*

I.37 VĪTARĀGAVIṢAYAṂ VĀ CITTAM

Vīta = *free (from)*
Rāga = *attachment*
Viṣayaṁ = *objects of the senses*
Vā = *or*
Cittam = *mind-stuff*

Or By Concentrating On A Great Soul's Mind, Which Is Totally Freed From Attachment To Sense Objects, The Devotee's Mind (Gets Stabilized).

This verse seems to be suggesting that if we can't find that supreme detachment ourselves, we think of a Being who represents that to us. Again this *sūtra* reminds us of the power of the mind. Whatever it focuses on can be brought forth into manifestation.

The focus can be whatever our symbol of a role model is, one that we would aspire to. This could take the form of a friend, teacher or someone we may have met who seemed to exemplify traits and characteristics that we perceive as unattached and free from desire. There are beautiful symbols and forms in many religions that are inspiring. There is not just one way, one form, or belief.

Now Patañjali suggests that one attains the state of *samādhi* by focusing on the mind or essence of a Great Soul, who is free from desire. This can be a teacher, *guru*, saint, sage or any figurehead of any world religion that you find inspirational. This person can be either living or non-living. It can be one who has achieved immortality in the collective psyche of humankind.

Many find inspiration from those who have transcended worldly desire through the memory of great ones such as Ramana Maharshi, Rama Krishna, Paramāhansa Yogānanda, Jesus the Christ, His Holiness The Dalai Lama, Mahatma Gandhi, Saint Teresa of Avila and more currently Mother Teresa, now canonized as a saint. Saint Francis can also be a symbol of total detachment, even relinquishing attachment to wearing clothes.

There is no prescribed form that is suggested, only that which represents the desireless qualities of non-attachment. It could be the author of a book, or someone you have met in your life who uplifts your heart and brings peace to your soul simply by thinking about them.

There are so many forms we may choose to help us cultivate that essence of non-attachment to worldly desires including Universal expansion of the mind into the vast reaches of outer space and the formless qualities of the Eternal Cosmic Vibration.

EXERCISE:
Discuss or Journal on the following questions:
1) *Who are those Beings in your life that bring you solace whenever you think of them?*
2) *Who are those you may read or hear about that represent the utmost of detachment, faith and compassion?*
3) *What are the qualities, you yourself would want to aspire to?*
4) *Who inspires you in just thinking about them?*

I.38 SVAPNANIDRĀJÑĀNĀLAMBANAṂ VĀ

***Svapna** = dream*
***Nidrā** = deep sleep*
***Jñāna** = becoming acquainted*
***Ālambana** = to hold attention*
***Vā** = or*

(Or) By Concentrating On An Experience Had During Dreams Or Deep Sleep.

There are times we may feel as we are taken to the great halls of learning and are taught during our sleep. There may also be times when we feel the touch and words of wisdom from invisible Divine masters who come towards us during the sleeping hours to teach and expand our consciousness beyond the earthly experiences.

In conscious dreaming we can take charge of our lives through our dreams.

If we focus on those dreams during the waking hours it is ever uplifting, leading to that state of *Yogaś Citta Vṛtti Nirodhaḥ*. It seems as if every *sūtra* is based on helping us to come into that state of what Vyasa calls "stability" and what we may call "stillness."

In dreams, we have no cognition or awareness of the external world. Like sleep, dreams are a deeply internal experience. When we have an elevating or creative thought in a dream, or even a "good" feeling, it is recommended that upon waking, we use that as an uplifting focal point of contemplation. As we learn to recall the dream from memory, eventually even in the

dream, we might be able to cultivate the awareness that we are dreaming. Whatever the pleasant or uplifting memory of the dream, it can eventually be taken into the waking state and used as a form of concentration.
It helps to keep a dream journal, making note of anything remembered about the dream upon waking. There are prophetic dreams where in the sleep state, we may slip into a future dimension where events yet to come are revealed through the dream. There are dreams that seem more real than the events in our waking life. There are dreams that may appear as nightmares, bringing our deep latent fears up for healing.

In sleep, the conscious mind is subdued by the subconscious, which becomes more active. Consciously dreaming, being aware that we are dreaming, helps us gain greater understanding of what is lying in the depths of our subconscious mind. Any undesirable images can be positively transformed when we are aware that we are dreaming. Like anything else, this requires awareness and practice.

Dreams can be a distorted reflection of life's events. In conscious dreaming we can take charge of our lives through our dreams. Rather than letting the events in our dreams control us, we learn to move the dream in an inspiring and uplifting direction. Some people feel helpless and powerless to make changes in the dream-like state. However, through practice one can learn to move the dream in a desired direction. This gives greater clarity, understanding and mastery of situations in one's life and helps subdue the turbulent waves (*vṛttis*) of the mind.

There may be times when we feel the touch and words of wisdom from invisible Divine masters who come towards us during the sleeping hours to teach and expand our consciousness beyond the earthly experiences

I.39 YATHĀBHIMATA DHYĀNĀD VĀ

Yatha *= as, in which manner*
Abhimata *= per choice or desire, agreeableness*
Dhyānat *= from meditating*
Vā *= or*

Or, By Meditating On Anything One Chooses That Is Elevating.

In this first chapter, Patañjali gives yet another way in which the aspirant can realize the state of *Yogaś Citta Vṛtti Nirodhaḥ*. If it is difficult to practice the previous suggestions, he uses again and again the word "Or." This little conjunction signifies that there is more than one way to attain the stillness of mind and in turn realize the *samādhi* states.

What is so wonderful about *yoga* is that instead of expecting the aspirant to adapt to scripture, the scripture of the *Yoga Sūtras* seem to adapt to the natural inclinations of the student. In so doing, we go with the grain of our nature, rather than struggling against it.

After giving many alternatives, in this *sūtra* Patañjali gives the ultimate suggestion on how to attain the desired state of *Yogaś Citta Vṛtti Nirodhaḥ*, "Or by meditating on anything one chooses that is elevating." Wow! What freedom! We don't have to hammer ourselves into what can be a constricting belief system. We are free to choose whatever person or symbol that is elevating to us. It can be a deity or perhaps we may find our inspiration and stillness of mind by reflecting upon a sunrise or sunset, the sun, moon and stars. It might take the form of the beauty of a flower, or the unconditional love of a pet. That elevating symbol may be the vastness of an ocean, a waterfall, the unwavering stability of a tree, the innocence of a child or the caress of the wind. And sometimes, we might even find our thoughts elevated by the one who lives closest to us in our own home.

That Elevating Symbol May Be the Vastness of an Ocean, a Waterfall, the Unwavering Stability of a Tree, the Innocence of a Child or the Caress of the Wind.

EXERCISE

Discuss or Journal on the following questions:

1) *What is elevating to you?*
2) *What is it that uplifts your spirit when you feel the weight of the world is pulling or pushing you down?*
3) *What is it that you may think about that brings you back to the remembrance of that Divine spirit that pervades all particles of creation?*

Note: Throughout the four chapters of the sūtras, Patañjali gives a myriad of ways to still the mind in order to come into a desired state of samādhi. There are numerous references throughout this ancient text as to what we might today call "positive thinking." Thousands of years ago, seers understood the power of thought and its manifestation. Today, it is known in the "New Thought" movement as "Thoughts held in mind produce after their kind." This message is not new as will be seen throughout the sūtras that are over two thousand years old.

I.40 PARAMĀṆU PARAMAMAHATTVĀNTO'SYA VAŚĪKĀRAḤ

Paramāṇu = *primal atom, smallest*
Parama = *greatest*
Mahattva = *magnitude*
Antah = *end, extension*
Asya = *his/her*
Vaśīkāraḥ = *mastery*

Gradually One's Mastery In Contemplation Extends From The Primal Atom To The Greatest Magnitude.

Patañjali suggests here that we focus our mind on the atom, the smallest particle of our material world as well on the magnitude of the greatest. If the mind dwells between these two polarities, it is suggested that one gains mastery in bringing the mind under control. There's that word again, "control." Perhaps we might find another word such as "stability" or "unwavering stillness" or whatever one chooses.

This *sūtra* reminds me of Gaṇeśa, the elephant God of good fortune and remover of material and spiritual obstacles. Gaṇeśa with his giant body and belly represents the macrocosm. The vehicle that he rides upon is a tiny mouse. The mouse represents the microcosm. Together, they represent the interdependency and movement from the micro to macrocosm.

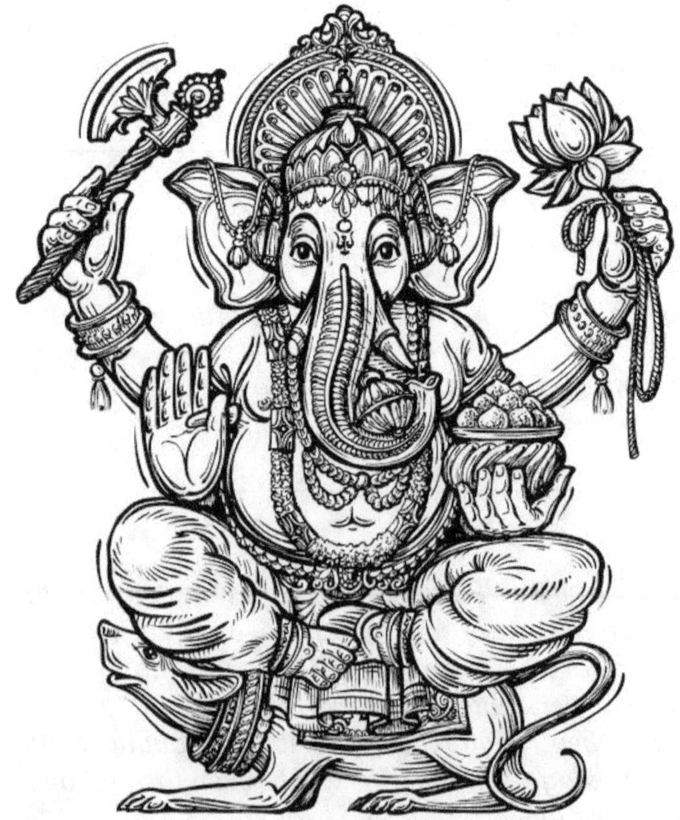

It is suggested that we focus on the concept of the *tanmatra* that is the minute atom or monad, and the subtlest of gross elements. At the same time, if we let the mind soar to whatever our macrocosmic concepts of the Universe might be, we create a powerful equalized tension between these two points. When this happens, the mind comes into equilibrium with balanced insight of a one-pointed mind. This is known in this *sūtra* as *samāpatti.* In this state, according to Swami Hariharānanda, one can reach the state of *asaṃprajñāta samādhi* , which is the "seedless" and most profound stage of *samādhi* that is beyond form.

We Focus Our Mind on the Atom,
the Small Particle of Our Material World ...
At the Same Time, If We Let the Mind Soar to Whatever Our
Macrocosmic Concepts of the Universe Might Be, We Create a
Powerful Equalized Tension Between These Two Points.

I.41 KṢĪṆA VṚTTER ABHIJĀTASYEVA MAṆER GRAHĪTṚ GRAHAṆA GRĀHYEṢU TATSTHA TADAÑJANATĀ SAMĀPATTIḤ

Kṣīṇa = *totally weakened, waned or dwindled*
Vṛtter = *modifications*
Abhijāta = *of natural pureness, of flawless*
Iva = *like, as if*
Maṇeh = *crystal*
Grahītṛ = *knower*
Grahaṇa = *knowledge*
Grāhyeṣu = *in knowledge (and)*
Tad = *by that*
Stha = *similar, being on or in*
Tad = *on that*
Añjanatā = *assuming the color of any near object*
Samāpattiḥ = *samādhi , balanced state, coincidence*

Just As The Naturally Pure Crystal Assumes Shapes And Colors Of Objects Placed Near It, So The Yogi's Mind With Its Totally Weakened Modifications (*Vṛttis*) Becomes Clear And Balanced And Attains The State Devoid Of Differentiation Between Knower, Knowable And Knowledge. This Culmination Of Meditation Is Known As *Samādhi*

This *sūtra* is a mouthful! Basically, it is speaking of the mind that is only partially quiet or still. This is a state where the modifications of the waves of the mind, known as *vṛttis*, are not as turbulent in their fluctuations. However, the waves are not totally still but existing in what Patañjali calls a "weakened" state. It does not mean the mind is weakened, but only the waves or modifications that arise *within* the field of the mind (*citta*) are becoming minimal and less distracting.

Whatever We Think We Become

This *sūtra*, like many, refers back to the 2nd and 3rd verses in this chapter. Here Patañjali speaks of the aspirant who is focusing on an object. Like a beautiful crystal, whatever object is placed on or near it, the crystal or gem will take on the tinge of whatever object is near it. Could this mean that whatever we focus on, we can take on the color or qualities of that object?

Vyasa supports this when he says, "Likewise when the mind is occupied with a liberated soul the mind displays the nature of such a soul." This is a powerful statement bringing the aspirant back to previous *sūtras*, which say in a variety of classical ways, "whatever we think we become." This theme keeps reoccurring, not only in this first chapter but in the third chapter as well.

Swami Hariharānanda's commentaries help to clarify what could be a confusing *sūtra*, "The concentration attained in a habitually one-pointed mind is called engrossment or *samāpatti*."

Swamiji then comments on the differences of this engrossment, which becomes increasingly more complex. To one struggling with everyday matters in their life, his esoteric commentaries of this *sūtra* may seem a bit "over the head." Perhaps by my saying this, you might want to read them, if only out of curiosity.

IN ĀSANA

It helps to observe our thoughts during the practice of *āsana*. The practices are very powerful. Whatever our thoughts at the time of entering into a pose, holding it and then exiting the pose makes that thought more powerful. If we can practice with our breath, it will help bring the mind to one point. As we move in this concentrated state in a continuous flow without interruption of thought, we can enter into *samāpatti* or engrossment.

Whatever our thoughts at the time of entering into a pose, holding it and then exiting the pose makes that thought more powerful

I.42 TATRA ŚABDĀRTHA JÑĀNA VIKALPAIḤ SAṂKĪRṆĀ SAVITARKĀ

***Tatra** = there*
***Śabda** = sound, word, name*
***Artha** = meaning, object, form*
***Jñāna** = knowledge, idea*
***Vikalpaiḥ** = assumptions, concept (these three)*
***Saṃkīrṇā** = mixed up*
***Savitarkā** = with deliberation*

The *Samādhi* In Which Name, Form And Knowledge Of Them Is Mixed Is Called *Savitarkā Samādhi* , Or *Samādhi* With Deliberation

The word engrossment is another name for *samādhi.* Since the name of this chapter is *samādhi pāda*, you will find that most of the emphasis is upon how to achieve that state. There are so many experiences and states of *samādhi* that Swami Hariharānanda covers in his text. This particular *sūtra* discusses a particular *samādhi* known as *savitarkā samāpatti.*

In ancient times, the term *tarkā* referred to "thought with the help of words." The word *vitarka* mentioned in this *sūtra*, is a particular kind of *tarkā*. Since *samādhi and* knowledge are considered to be inseparable, any knowledge acquired in *samādhi* is *vitarka* and it is known as *savitarkā samādhi* .

Knowledge attained in a particular state of concentration based on words is known as *savitarkā samāpatti.* This has three parts; 1) hearing the name 2) recalling the image attached to that name 3) and bringing forth knowledge of an object associated with that name.

To help understand this, Swami Satchidānanda uses the example of a dog and Swami Hariharānanda uses the image of a cow. When we hear the verbal sound of cow or dog, we bring to the mind, an image of the animal from our imagination (*vikalpa*) that is stored in our memory (*smṛti*).

When our imagination is triggered by the word cow or dog, we then automatically think of all we know about the animal. The cow gives milk, butter, cheese; it is a docile creature, etc. When we hear dog, our imagination and memory will pull up an image and then our knowledge of that dog based on our experiences that are either negative or positive; a dog tried to bite me once and I am afraid of dogs; or, my dog is my best friend, he loves me unconditionally.

Of course, in this particular *samādhi,* the intent is not to focus on cows or dogs even though they are wonderful animals. The main purpose of *savitarkā samāpatti* is to gain knowledge of the *tattvas*, which are the elements that lead to the knowledge of *prakṛti*, the divine earth principle of creation. This particular form of engrossment or *samādhi* , according to Swami Hariharānanda "leads to the development of detachment, leading gradually to the attainment of liberation."

I.43 SMṚTI PARIŚUDDHAU SVARŪPA ŚUNYEVĀRTHA MĀTRA NIRBHĀSĀ NIRVITARKĀ

Smṛti *= memory*
Pariśuddhau *= upon utmost purification*
Svarūpa *= its own nature, own form*
Śunya *= empty*
Iva *= as if*
Artha *= object*
Mātra *= only*
Nirbhāsā *= shining*
Nirvitarkā *= without deliberation*

When The Memory Is Well Purified, Devoid Of The Distinction Of Name And Quality, This Is *Nirvitarkā Samādhi,* Or *Samādhi* Without Deliberation.

> *Nirvitarkā would be knowledge gained without the help of words and their associations.*

Now we come to *nirvitarkā samādhi.* Since the term *vitarka* is associated with words in the recall of an object, *nirvitarkā* is its opposite. *Nir* would mean to negate the following verb of *vitarka*. Thus, *nirvitarkā* would be knowledge gained without the help of words and their associations. *Nirvitarkā samāpatti* is the simultaneous fusion of the three steps of *savitarkā*, mentioned in the previous *sūtra*. It is the collective retention and a fusion of consciousness of the *yogin* with any object of contemplation.

Swami Hariharānanda compares *nirvitarkā* with *savitarkā*. "A state of retention of impressions collected during concentration is *nirvitarkā samāpatti* and the recollection of such impressions with the help of words is *savitarkā samāpatti*."

In *nirvitarkā* there is no memory, recollection (*smṛti)*, no images (*vikalpa*), there is only the fusion beyond words, memory and imagination. A *yogin* in this state is like the moth that consumes itself in the flame and is immersed fully in the Divine Consciousness. This is the ultimate state of *gnana yoga*.

The state of *savitarkā samāpatti*, could be compared to *bhakti* a devotional expression of the nightingale singing its song and weeping for the rose. While it longs for that union, it continues to maintain distance and separation from its beloved so it can savor the experience of worshiping the Divine and recalling it after periodic glimpses of that Union.

> *In savitarkā, there is knowledge of the form,*
> *and the words and memories around the form*
> *but there is still separation.*
> *This could be compared to bhakti a devotional expression*
> *of the nightingale singing its song*
> *and weeping for the rose.*

Nirvitarkā is *samādhi* without deliberation of memory and imagination. There is no name (*sva*) or form (*rūpa*). It is devoid of reflective consciousness even forgetting that "I am knowing." In *nirvitarkā samāpatti* the subject and object of contemplation fuse into a most desired meditative state known as *nirvitarkā samādhi* .

IN ĀSANA

We can practice these *samādhis* in *āsana*. The posture *Jānu Śīrsāsana*, the one-legged forward bend would be an example. When bending forward to bring head to knee, bend from the hips rather than waist and offer belly to thigh as if offering yourself to the Divine while dwelling in the extended leg.

In *savitarkā*, there is knowledge of the form, and the words and memories around the form but there is still separation like the nightingale serenading the rose. But eventually, that separation may dissolve as you begin to close the gap between the upper and lower body fusing the two into the *One*, like the moth consuming itself in the magnificence of the flame. This fusion could be considered to be the state of *nirvitarkā samādhi.*

I.44 ETAYAIVA SAVICĀRĀ NIRVICĀRA CA SŪKṢMAVIṢAYĀ VYĀKHYĀTĀ

Etaya *= in the same way*
Iva *= indeed*
Savicārā *= reflective*
Nirvicāra *= super non-reflective*
Ca *= and*
Sūkṣma *= subtle*
Viṣaya *= objects*
Vyākhyātā *= are explained*

In The Same Way, Both *Savicārā* (Reflective) And *Nirvicāra* (Super Or Non-Reflective *Samādhi)*, Which Are Practiced Upon Subtle Objects, Are Explained.

Take a deep breath. Even if you have had brief glimpses of these *samādhi* states, when words attempt to explain them, it can be a bit confusing.

Now, Patañjali goes more deeply into the next two stages of *samādhi, savicārā* and *nirvicāra.*

The previous two sūtras addressed concepts of *savitarkā* and *nirvitarkā samādhi. Savitarkā* and *nirvitarkā* are said to relate to gross elements and *savicārā* and *Nirvicāra* are related to subtle elements. The term *vicāra* relates to subtle objects.

According to the translations of Swami Hariharānanda, "*Savicārā* is a reflective *samādhi* that takes place in the gross forms of the elements that are conditioned by space, time and causation." This means that in *savicārā*, knowledge *is* confined to a particular space.

In *nirvicāra samādhi,* however, it is the opposite. Knowledge is not conditioned by space, time and causation. *Nirvicāra is not* limited to the present time only but extends to the past, present and future simultaneously. This is a state of engrossment where the three concepts of time become superimposed upon one another and where knowledge *is not* confined by a particular space.

Nirvicāra Samādhi
Patañjali defines *nirvicāra* as supra-reflective engrossment that pertains to the unmanifested *prakṛti.* This is a very subtle state where atomic and sub-atomic particles are realized in their elemental form of light, sound, touch, smell and taste known as *tanmatras.* In this state, it is as if a veil had been removed. Instead of seeing solid objects as distinguishable from one another, they become moving waves and particles in space that comprise our third dimensional reality — or unreality. In this state, we perceive the subtlety of the *tanmatras* that give our world form.

When we see beyond the form, the world as we know transforms into vibratory frequencies of energy and light where it is difficult to perceive one object or form from another. This experience would be the state of *nirvicāra samādhi.*

Nirvitarkā (in the previous *sūtra*) is free from ideas created by the imagination (*vikalpa*). So too is *nirvicāra*. When either *nirvitarkā* and *nirvicāra samādhi* is attained as Swami Hariharānanda says, "material possessions like wealth, family, etc., cease to have any charm and they always appear as mere combinations of light, sound, touch, smell, etc."

In *nirvicāra samādhi* like *nirvitarkā*, that which appears "real" becomes illusory. This is the un-manifested state of *prakṛti* (nature) where solidity of material objects dissolve back into their elements of *tanmatras*. Words and concepts no longer bind our consciousness in the illusion of solidity but go beyond to show the minutest particles that comprise creation.

Nirvicāra is similar to *nirvitarkā* in that they both transcend words, concepts and the recall of memory and imagination. In these states of *samādhi,* solidity of material objects and the words used to describe them drop away.

Savicārā Samādhi

Now let's look at *savicārā samādhi.* Swami Hariharānanda says, "*Savicārā* engrossment is conditioned by words, objects and their knowledge all mixed together; and is consequently affected by space, time and causation."

Savicārā, like *savitarkā*, is conditioned by words, objects and their knowledge. Swami Hariharānanda comments, "*Tanmatra* is not the only object of *savicārā samāpatti*. Other subtle objects like *ahaṁkāra* or mutative ego, *buddhi* or pure I-sense and un-manifest *prakṛti* or constituent principles in equilibrium (three *guṇas*) also serve as objects of *savicārā samāpatti.*"

Swami Hariharānanda speaks of the un-manifested *prakṛti* being the potential state of all phenomena and says it cannot be an object of meditation because it cannot be seen or apprehended. He says "Hence there cannot be any *nirvicāra* engrossment on *prakṛti. Prakṛtilaya* (absorption in *prakṛti*) means dissolution of *citta* into its causal substance but it is not *samāpatti.* However, a *yogin* whose mind has once merged into *prakṛti* can have *savicārā* knowledge of *prakṛti*. This is *savicārā samāpatti* (engrossment) on *prakṛti.*"

Note: Even if we have had glimpses of a few of these states, it is still confusing to put those experiences into words. To understand these sūtras and the elaborate and esoteric commentaries by Swami Hariharānanda it is important to contemplate upon their meaning through meditation. After all, that is what these sūtras in Chapter I are based upon. As we are able to delve deeper into our yoga practices, these sūtras on savitarkā, nirvitarkā, savicārā and nirvicāra samādhi s may become an experience rather than an intellectual concept.

IN ĀSANA

There may be times in *āsana*, when we feel as if one part of our body is fusing into another. If we can reach a point of stillness of mind within the pose where the breath is no longer a distraction, we may come into a transcended state of the un-manifested *prakṛti*. In one pose, we can merge from the *savicārā* into the *nirvicāra* state where the material world and the solidity of our body dissolve into a subtle field of atomic and subatomic particles. The only thing that can hold us back from this experience is fear.

> *Words and concepts no longer bind our consciousness in the illusion of solidity but go beyond to show the minutest particles that comprise creation*

When entering into an immersion of consciousness in a *samādhi* state, in any pose, if we do not feel the support of the material world, the ego (*ahaṁkāra*) can become frightened of its own annihilation. As we continue our practices, we develop greater faith, physical and spiritual stamina and courage that helps us to transcend our fears as we surrender to that Universal essence. Here in the *sūtras*, it is called *Īśvara praṇidhāna.*

If we can practice *āsana* as an offering to the Divine, the benefits are multi-faceted. Not only does this humble our ego, transforming its energy into realization of the Divine but through this practice, we learn greater trust in the invisible guidance that is always present and protecting us. It restores and strengthens our faith in a power greater than our own, allowing our consciousness to dive into the deeper and more expansive states of consciousness without fear.

Each pose of *yoga* is considered to be a *mudrā*. *Mu* in this instance means form and *dra* from *drav* means "to flow along with form." These are the gestures of the mind expressing itself through the movements of the body. *Āsana* is a *mudrā*. There are said to be 84 basic poses and a thousand variations on each. The word thousand in the eastern cultures means infinite. Therefore, there are infinite ways in which the mind can express itself through the body. Preparation for the most expanded forms of *samādhi* may require a new spatial awareness. *Āsanas* help us to do this.

An example would be when at first we take an inverted pose, there may be a sense of fear. But as our mind gets more accustomed to the pose, the fear will gradually drop away building trust and even faith in our self. Fears ultimately relate, not just to death, but "fear of the unknown." *Āsana* variations give ever-new opportunities to move from the known to the unknown. Eventually, the unknown becomes the known and so forth.

For instance, for years we may have had a fear of the headstand. We finally master it and overcome our fear. But one day, the teacher asks us to drop backwards from the headstand and new fears may arise. This gives us a new opportunity to face another fear. Here again, we learn to move from the known to the unknown and slowly learn to trust in our new spatial awareness that expands with each new variation and each new situation.

Therefore, *āsana* can prepare us to enter into the deeper and more expanded states of consciousness where objects of solidity and familiarity dissolve into a sea of moving atomic particles and subatomic particles. We cannot enter into these "higher" forms of *samādhi,* unless we are prepared to totally surrender, without fear, into the unfamiliar and unexplored regions of *samādhi.* This requires total trust and faith in a power far greater than our own. It seems as if the *sūtra* verses of *Īśvara praṇidhāna* prepare us for these later *sūtras* in this chapter.

Āsana with breath can bring up to the surface of our mind, latent or hidden impressions embedded within our subconscious mind. The practice of *āsana* brings these to the surface of the mind for healing and releasing.

I.45 SŪKṢMA VIṢAYATVAM CĀLIṄGA PARYAVASĀNAM

***Sūkṣma** = subtle*
***Viṣayatvaṃ** = objectiveness*
***Ca** = and*
***Aliṅga** = without mark, indefinable, unmanifest prakṛti*
***Paryavasānam** = end only at, all the way up to*

Subtlety Pertaining To Objects Culminates In A-Liṅga Or The Unmanifested.

"There is nothing as subtle as the unmanifested," Vyasa's commentaries say, "but the subtlety of *puruṣa* is not the same kind as that of the unmanifested. It is said that subtlety has reached its limit in *pradhāna* or *prakṛti* (which is the state of equilibrium of the three *guṇas,* or constituent principles."

Here again, the *sūtra* supports the second *sūtra* for when the three *guṇas* come into equilibrium with one another, the mind is automatically in *Yogaś Citta Vṛtti Nirodhaḥ* and then the seer and seen become One, or realize the Oneness that already is.

According to Swami Hariharānanda, "The term *liṅga* is that which terminates or merges into its cause." When there is a short "A" in front of the verb, it reverses the meaning. So *a-liṅga* would mean it has no cause. It is that which has not merged into any other substance. *Pradhāna* and *prakṛti* are considered to be *a-liṅga*. This would be the unmanifest *prakṛti,* nature.

Swamiji continues his commentaries, "The *tanmatras* are the minutest sensations of subtle objects received by the senses. The external cause of such perception is the ego of the Great Divine Mind known as *Bhūtadi*."

Let's leave it at that. The commentaries speak of *puruṣa* and *prakṛti* intimating that *puruṣa* does not suffer the changes that *prakṛti* does. But they say that *prakṛti* is changed into *mahat*, the cosmic mind that is ultimately the child of both *puruṣa* and *prakṛti*.

Again, these later *sūtras* in Chapter I seem to appeal to an intense student, perhaps an *intense*, intense student. But Chapter II is something all aspirants will understand and the practices are tangible and practical. This chapter becomes more and more subtle as the *sūtras* unfold, one into the next.

I.46 TĀ EVA SABĪJAḤ SAMĀDHIḤ

***Tā** = they*
***Eva** = indeed*
***Sabījaḥ** = with seed*
***Samādhi** = contemplation*

Each Of The Above Kinds Of *Samādhi Are Sabīja* (With Seed), Which Could Bring One Back Into Bondage Or Mental Disturbances.

The preceding *sūtras* that address the various states of *samādhi are* all considered to be "with seed." The ideal state of consciousness to the *yogin* would be that which is "seedless." In Sanskrit this is known as *nirbīja* (without seed). *Sabīja* and *nirbīja*, the *samādhi* states of consciousness with seed and without seed are mentioned again in Chapter III, *Vibhuti Pada* (III:8).

When a *samādhi* state is tinged with imagination, memory, and the I-sense of the ego, it still has "seeds" of attachment. According to *yoga* scriptures, this means that when one dies, the soul, still fettered with earthly attachments, will reincarnate back into this 3rd dimensional plane. This *sūtra* speaks of this as "bondage" or "mental disturbances."

The mental disturbance here relates to the mental modification of the three *guṇas* that manifest through the *vṛttis*, the mind waves. Their oscillating interaction gives form to what we call life. However, this life is lived in a very limited dimension that is called *maya* or *avidyā*.
The verb *ma* means to measure and the suffix *ya* means *yeah, really do it!* Then *maya* would mean an extreme form of measurement that implies distance and separation.

The word *maya* is more of a Vedantic term while *avidyā* is a *yogic* term used here in the *sūtras*. The letter "A" means to negate and *vidyā* is seeing, piercing through. *Avidyā* would then mean, we are really *no*t piercing through or we are really *not* seeing.

We may have periodic *samādhi* experiences. But if they still hold the seeds of unresolved attachments, or any other residue within the hidden vaults of our psyche, we are not fully liberated and free from *avidyā*. From the scriptures this means that upon death, the soul may reach one of the heavenly abodes of a celestial plane. Even though for many this is a desired state, for the *yogin*, it is not.

Patañjali in Chapter II, addresses the intricate patterns of *karma*, its negative and positive influences and how *karma* impacts our present existence and future lives.

It is believed that when a person dies after attaining a "lower" *samādhi* state "with seed," they may dwell in a beautiful and blissful realm of consciousness that is filled with forms of angels, *Devas* and other light beings. Because they have not reached the most expanded form of *samādhi,* they will linger in this seed form of *samādhi* consciousness for a designated period of time. Time has a different connotation in these subtle states of consciousness. A thousand years on earth may seem like a moment in the celestial spheres.

If one has not reached the "seedless" form of *samādhi,* it is believed that when their positive merits, previously accrued here on earth, run out, it is time for them to reincarnate back into the earth plane.

This can sound discouraging for one seeking total liberation. However, it is hopeful to know that whatever lessons we have accumulated in the refinement of our own evolutionary process in our life on earth, remains with us during our cyclic transitions.

However, that does not mean that when returning to the earth plane, one is not subjected to the turbulence of the mental modifications (*vṛttis*). It does not mean that one can return free of the disturbances of the oscillation of the constituents of nature known as the three *guṇas*, inertia, activity and equanimity.

Patañjali says in a myriad of ways, that the purpose of *yoga* is to bring the *guṇas* into balanced equilibrium. When this happens, the oscillations of the mind cease and one comes into the desired state of stillness (I:2)

The classic intent of *yogins* however, is not "to go to heaven", but to go beyond into the nameless and formless spheres of consciousness from which there is no return to the earth plane. These *samādhi* states are discussed in great detail in Chapter III. There are mystics, known and unknown throughout the ages who have made a conscious choice not to enter into full immersion with the Divine. They have done this in order to return to this earth plane as way-showers for others to understand the nature of existence and how to transcend suffering while in this world. In Buddhism they are called *bodhisattvas*.

Sri Aurobindo Gosh believed that after experiencing the *samādhi* state, instead of trying to get out of this world, we may choose to stay in it and use our transcendental awareness to help transform this world into the replica of the worlds we are trying "to get to."

This *sūtra* brings to mind an amusing story of two monks sitting on the side of a road, doing their spiritual disciplines and practices year after year. One day, Sage Nārada walked by and the monks stopped him. "Oh great Sage, where are you going?" He stopped, looked at the two monks and said, "I am going to *Vaikuntha* to see God. *Vaikuntha* is the Hindu term for heaven or the abode of Lord Vishnu. "Oh," replied one monk excitedly. "Can you ask God for me how many more lives I have left on this earthly plane?" The other little monk humbly and quietly asked, "Can you ask God for me too?" Sage Nārada agreed and continued his journey.

After a few years, the great sage returned from the heavenly abode, went down the road where he found the monks. The first monk asked, "Did you see God?" Sage Nārada nodded saying, "Yes. Yes, I did." The monk, breathless with anticipation asked, "Did he say how many more lives I have to live?"

The sage replied, "Yes. He said you have four more lives to live." The monk was livid with rage and began jumping up and down on his *mala* beads yelling, "Four more lives? After all the *sādhana* I have done faithfully for all these years and he says I have four more lives." He was furious.

The other little monk whispered, "Did God say how many more lives I have to live." The illustrious sage pointed to the leaves on the giant Banyan tree sheltering them. "Do you see the leaves of this tree? That is how many more lives you have to live." The little monk began jumping up and down shouting with joy. "How wonderful! Thousands of more lives to serve the Divine." As the story goes, he was instantly transformed into the highest *samādhi* state from where one does not have to return to the earth plane.

EXERCISE:

Journal and Discuss on the Following Questions:

1) *What does this story mean to you?*
2) *What do you think and feel about the seed form of samadhi.*

Chapter III goes into the seed and seedless aspects of consciousness.

3) *Without reading ahead, what do you think the "seeds" are within your own consciousness that may be your soul's anchor to this earth plane?*

I.47 NIRVICĀRA VAIŚĀRADYE 'DHYĀTMA PRASĀDAḤ

Nirvicāra *= non-reflective*
Vaiśāradye *= pure, lucid*
Adhyātma *= supreme Self*
Prasādaḥ *= shine, clear*

In The Purity Of *Nirvicāra Samādhi,* The Pure Self Shines

Here Patañjali discusses *nirvicāra samādhi,* that is the most expansive of the four *samādhis* mentioned in this chapter: *savitarkā, nirvitarkā, savicārā* and *nirvicāra.*

It is hoped the following commentaries by Vyasa will help to better understand this *sūtra.*

"When impurities, which shade the illuminating nature of *buddhi* are removed, there is a transparent flow of quiescence free from the taints of *rajas* and *tamas* and this is called attainment of proficiency. When the *yogin* gets such proficiency in *nirvicāra* concentration he achieves purity in his inner instrument of reception from which he gets the power of knowing things as they are simultaneously without any sequence of time, and in all their aspects. In other words, he acquires the clear light of knowledge through powers of realization.

It has been said in this connection in the *Mahābhārata* (the great epic of India), "As a man on the hilltop sees a man on the plains, so one having ascended the palace of knowledge and becoming free from sorrow now sees others who are suffering."

Note: It is amazing how Patañjali weaves back and forth in all the chapters, saying the same thing in a variety of ways. This, no doubt relates to the nine types of students and methods of learning. (I:22)

> *"As a man on the hilltop sees a man on the plains,*
> *so one having ascended the palace of knowledge*
> *and becoming free from sorrow*
> *now sees others who are suffering."*
>
> *The Mahabharata*

I.48 ṚTAMBHARĀ TATRA PRAJÑĀ

Ṛtam *= absolute truth*
Bharā *= bearing*
Tatra *= there*
Prajñā *= wisdom consciousness*

The Knowledge That Is Gained In That State Is Called Ṛtambharā (Filled With Truth).

The *Ṛ* in *rtam* is pronounced *ri* which means to rise upwards. And *bharā* is bearing. In *ṛtambhar*ā we are rising upwards and bearing or holding the Truth. *Ṛtambharā* is a beautiful word filled with rhythm and when it is coupled with *prajñā*, it is even more powerful. *Pra* means to bring forth and *jñā* is wisdom. So in *ṛtambharā prajñā* we might loosely define it as "Rising upward bearing or upholding the Truth in bringing forth the wisdom."

What does it mean in *ṛtambharā*, "To Be Filled With Truth?" *Ṛtambha*rā, defined as unalloyed Truth is in essence, a "seedless" *samādhi*. As Vyasa says, "It retains and sustains truth along with no misconception."

Patañjali explains this further in the following *sūtra*.

I.49 ŚRUTĀNUMĀNA PRAJÑĀBHYĀM ANYA VIṢAYĀ VIŚEṢĀRTHATVĀT

Śruta *= study of scriptures (scriptures are heard)*
Anumāna *= inference*
Prajñābhyām *= from the knowledge of both*
Anya *= different (totally)*
Viṣayā *= domain (truth)*
Viśeṣa *= special*
Arthatvat *= from its significance, from its purposefulness*

This Special Truth Is Totally Different From Knowledge Gained By Hearing, Study Of Scripture or Inference.

This *sūtra* again is unfolding from the previous one in reference to *ṛtambharā prajñā*, (filled with the wisdom of truth). In *ṛtambharā prajñā*, one transcends limitations of the portals of the human mind to have a direct experience of the

Eternal. It does not come from reading, attending classes or hearing about God. It is one's own direct inner communion with the Divine.

> *Ṛtambharā Prajñā is not an intellectual concept to be grasped by the human mind, but is a direct experiential communion with God.*

Ṛtambharā prajñā is a direct experience of *samādhi* state that goes beyond the experience of others such as teachers, masters, saints, sages and theologians. It is a state that goes beyond reading and listening to scriptures that is known as "inference from others."

It is not an intellectual concept to be grasped by the human mind, but is a direct experiential communion with God. Sometimes, we rely on the experiences of others until we have our own experience. There are times, when the experience of another supports our own inner revelations. And there are times when the inference of scriptures seems to verify the validity of our own inner experiences. This can give us greater faith and trust in ourselves so we cannot be shaken from that experience of Truth.

St. Teresa of Avila, Spain is a classic example of one who had the direct experience with God. When the church fathers deemed that her experience was not of God, but of the Devil, she stood up to them and refused to believe those who had not had the experience. Because she had the direct experience of God, nothing could shake her from that Truth.

Until we have our own inner *samādhi* experiences, it helps to hear and read of the great mystics throughout the ages who have been blessed by the invisible hand of the Eternal.

> *There are times, when the experience of another supports our own inner revelations. This can give us greater faith and trust in ourselves so we cannot be shaken from our experience of Truth.*

I.50 TAJJAḤ SAṂSKĀRO 'NYA SAṂSKĀRA PRATIBANDHĪ

***Tad** = that*
***Jaḥ** = born of, produced by*
***Saṃskāra** = subliminal impression*
***Anya** = other*
***Pratibandhī** = wipes out, replaces*

The Impressions Produced By This Samādhi Wipes Out All Other Impressions.

The impressions mentioned in this *sūtra* are known as *saṃskāras*, which are the latent impressions lying in the psyche of the subconscious mind. *(Saṃskāras are discussed in-depth in Chapter II.*)

Patañjali here mentions that in the state of *ṛtambharā prajñā* past impressions of delusion, attachment and anger, etc. would be "wiped out." In this *ṛtambharā prajñā samādhi* one becomes a realized soul, a *jivamukti*, who is liberated while living. *Jiva* means to live and *mukta* refers to release or liberate. In this state, one lives free of attachments, anger, aversion, etc. One has achieved *paravairāgya,* supreme detachment and they are liberated while in body. They live in service of others. Their presence on earth can lighten the atmospheric density of the planet. They are beyond the subliminal impressions or *saṃskāras* of the past. These former impressions no longer have any hold over them. In the *jivanmukti*, "seeds" of past impressions are scorched, never to sprout again. This would then be the *nirbīja* or "seedless" state of *samādhi*, known as *ṛtambharā prajñā samādhi.*

Jiva means to live and *mukta* refers to release or liberate.
In this *Ṛtambharā Prajñā Samadhi,* one becomes a Realized Soul, a *Jivamukti....*

"The imaginary world recedes from view and falls like a withered leaf and the soul (Jiva) remains like a fired grain, without the power of vegetation or reproduction."

- Yoga Vaśiṣṭha

What happens to such a mind?

I.51 TASYĀPI NIRODHE SARVA NIRODHĀN NIRBĪJAḤ SAMĀDHIḤ

***Tasya** = of that*
***Api** = even (also)*
***Nirodha** = upon being wiped out, upon the restraint*
***Sarva** = all*
***Nirodhān** = from being wiped out, due to restraint*
***Nirbījaḥ** = seedless*
***Samādhiḥ** = contemplation*

When This Impression Is Wiped Out, Every Impression Is Totally Wiped Out And There Is Nirbīja (Seedless) Samādhi.

At last! Patañjali has taken us through each verse as one folds into next. In this chapter, he explains the ultimate essence of why we are practicing *yoga*. In a logical sequence, he describes obstacles and the varying states of consciousness. It is so brilliantly designed where this last verse is supporting the 2nd and 3rd verses in the beginning of this chapter.

What happens in consciousness when the modifications (*vṛttis*) of the mind become still? As is said in this *sūtra* as in the previous one, all the impressions or *saṃskāras* of past and present are "wiped out."

This is the ultimate state of a seedless state of consciousness known as *samprajñāna samādhi.* When the knowledge of the *tattvas*, subtle elements are illumined through *samādhi* and are retained in a one-pointed mind, it is known as *samprajñāna*. When knowledge gained in this *samādhi* is eliminated (wiped out) it is a *nirbīja*, seedless state of *samādhi.*

When this happens the fluctuations (*vṛttis*) of the mind are totally arrested and the three *guṇas* come into perfect equilibrium. Then the Seer is regarded as pure and in turn, free from sorrow, the Seer is then liberated. In that state of liberation as mentioned in Verse 3, the Seer and Seen become One, or realize the Oneness that already is.

Thus ends the first Chapter of Patañjali's Yoga Sūtras Known as Samādhi Pada.

CHAPTER ONE SELF EVALUATION

1) What are the names of the four chapters of Patañjali's Yoga Sūtras?

Sanskrit	English
1.	1.
2.	2.
3.	3.
4.	4.

2) Why is the second sūtra the most important sūtra in Chapter One?

3) What are the Four Parts of Mind?

Sanskrit	English
1.	1.
2.	2.
3.	3.
4.	4.

4) What are the Five Non-Painful Mind Waves (*vṛttis*)?

Sanskrit	English
1.	1.
2.	2.
3.	3.
4.	4.
5.	5.

5) How are these *vṛttis* interacting at this time within your life?

CHAPTER ONE SELF EVALUATION

6) What are some various interpretations on the translation of *abhyāsa*? How do you experience sūtra II:12 in your *āsana* practice? In your life?

7) In Chapter One, Patañjali mentions obstacles to stilling the waves of the mind. What are those impediments that disturb the mind? How many are there and what are they called (in English)?

8) There are varying degrees of *samādhi* mentioned in Chapter One. Can you name three and describe them.

9) Patañjali gives many ways in Chapter One to still the waves of the mind. Which way or ways appeals to you the most? Why?

CHAPTER ONE SELF EVALUATION

10) Through your readings, journaling, discussions and homeplay throughout your journey in Chapter One of the Yoga Sūtras, what new insights, discoveries or changes have unfolded.... In your yoga practice? In your life?

Acknowledgments

It takes a village? There are no words to thank all of the *yoga* students who have listened patiently to my many talks on the *Yoga Sūtras* that I have given for the past 40 years. Finally, as they requested, these workbooks on the *Yoga Sūtras* are divided into four chapters that are now becoming available ... at long last.

My heart is filled with appreciation for those brave souls who have come forth to help me bring this version of the *Yoga Sūtras* into manifestation:

MIRA MURPHY, my daughter, who is an ayurvedic chef and a teacher of ayurveda and *yoga* workshops. She tirelessly sat by my side at the computer typing in my voluminous notes that went back in history to 1968 when I first began my studies into this infinite subject. One of the great miracles was that Mira could actually read my handwritten shorthand scribbles, and helped put them in order. She said she loved working on this project, feeling as I do that it is an honor to be able to speak, think and help write on this vast and timeless material.

Mira is the only one of my five children who is carrying on my work and developing her own work in teaching workshops in *yoga*, ayurveda and healing through foods. She is truly a *yogini* and healer who is illuminating the path of ayurveda and *yoga* for generations to come. Our hearts are ever connected.

ANN WAGONER, who 10 years ago came to Sedona to help me put my teachings into the written form. She saw, even before I did, that the legacy of *yoga* must be documented for future generations of teachers and students. Ann worked round the clock to help me organize five feet high paper piles and bring it into an order that gave a foundation for these chapters.

Years ago, Ann had the vision of recording question and answer sessions where she would ask well thought out questions on *yoga* and record my answers. Her unique way of asking questions would draw me into greater depths of myself in answering them.

Ann too felt it an honor to work on this project that seemed to plumb the depths of *yoga*, and how the *sūtras* directly applied to our *yoga* practice as well as to everyday life. She contacted publishers and looked into self-publishing, and out of this she was encouraged to start her own publishing company. Her grandfather was a publisher who helped Robert Frost among others, so she is now following her family's dharmic path, along with teaching ayurveda and *yoga*. She founded the Center for Ayurveda and Yoga Study in Portland, Oregon and serves as the president of the Oregon Yoga and Ayurveda Association.

I thank Ann for her vision and encouragement in continuing this project even while I was traveling and teaching. My heart is filled with love and thankfulness for Ann's help, guidance and vision.

GINNY BEAL — When the heart is full, the mouth is empty. It is so hard to convey a thankfulness that is beyond words. Ginny is that to me. She has supported me in my work for over 10 years now. She began by volunteering to organize *yoga* and *Yoga Sūtra* workshops nationally and internationally. In this project, Ginny took on the enormous task of editing. This was a time consuming task that she dedicated herself to completely. She said that it was helpful to read and edit Chapter 1 during challenging events that were unfolding in her own life.

Ginny too is a major part of the completion of this project. She has held the vision of the publication of my interpretation of the *Yoga Sūtras* for many years and is now editing and witnessing its completion chapter-by-chapter. She has organized my workshops, classes and retreats, interacting with many teachers in the broader *yoga* community. She has been studying and teaching *yoga* for many years and is dedicated to the future of *yoga* both nationally and globally.

CYNTHIA RUSSELL — A special thanks to Cynthia for using her talent and gifts of healing through music and mantra. Her knowledge of Sanskrit sounds and pronunciations has been invaluable. She volunteered to electronically insert the Sanskrit diacritical markings for accurate phonetic pronunciations. She has also transcribed my past recordings of classes and interviews. She is amazing in the evolvement of her classes of *yoga* and the healing vibration of sound. She has created a leading edge curriculum of Sanskrit sounds for healing body, mind and emotions. Cynthia also did the diacritical markings for my first book, *Yoga: The Practice of Myth and Sacred Geometry.*

CAROL LEVY — A special thanks to Carol who has helped me with the covers for all four chapters of the *Yoga Sūtras.* Carol is the founder and owner of Giraphics, a graphic and design company in Tyler, Texas, who understands the concepts of *yoga* in her everyday life. She has gone the extra mile to invest her time, interest and talent to create the covers for each chapter as well as charts. I cannot thank her enough for the time and energy she has invested in this project.

LAURA WEBBER has recently joined our team to help with spreading the word about my previous book and now the *Yoga Sūtras*. Laura, who is studying for a M.A. in Peace and Justice at the University of San Diego, is a teacher of *yoga* and will be applying the philosophy and psychology of *yoga* to her work in conflict resolution and social justice. Laura is dedicated to making the world a better place through the practice and deeper understanding of *yoga*.

Love,
Rama

Recommended Readings

***Yoga Philosophy of Patañjali,* by Samkhya Yogacharya Swami Hariharananda Aranya** (translated by P.N. Mukerji), State University of New York Press.

In 1971, when I was studying with Mr. B.K.S. Iyengar in India, he sent me to his personal bookseller to get this book. At the time, this was the book from which he drew much of his inspiration. After returning to the United States with a suitcase filled with these books for other *yoga* teachers, I opened the book to begin an in depth study of the *sūtras* and then quickly closed it. It was filled with Sanskrit terminology and esoteric commentaries that were far beyond my comprehension and understanding at the time. I promptly put it under the bed pillow in hopes that like Edgar Cayce, I could sleep on it and absorb some of its wisdom while I slept.

I immediately began the study of Sanskrit and after two years, I was awakened one night with the vibrational sounds of this ancient language filling the space of my mind. I opened the book and suddenly the *sūtras* as well as the commentaries were understandable. It was a moment in time where the great lineages that created and preserved these vast teachings were speaking and teaching through the pages. This version of the *sūtras* became my bible of *yoga* from that night on. The study never ends. Each time I make the leap into this beloved book, new glimmers of understandings continue to reveal themselves.

As we change, and unfold into new awareness over the years, perspectives and understandings of the *sūtras* can change also. Each time I open this book there are always new and inspirational insights, and a feeling of the presence of the masters who have created and preserved these teachings for generations to come.

This version of the *sūtras* is the most esoteric translation in the English language of this era. It vibrates with the pulse of the ancient heritage of the great masters of *yoga*. *Yoga Philosophy of Patañjali* is given original commentary by Vyasa, which has further commentary by Swami Hariharananda. P.N. Mukerji rendered it into English.

Today, several decades later, this version continues to inspire me. Whenever I open the book, it's like a communion with the ancient masters even beyond that of Patañjali, who compiled this great work thousands of years ago. He preserved the teachings of *yoga* in brief aphorisms that could be transmitted to future generations. This particular translation for me is like time travel into an ancient world of those who have cleared the path before us.

My lengthy commentaries are a humble attempt to help others understand how these teachings are applicable in our culture today, and weave into our *yoga* practices as well as our lives.

***Raja Yoga Sūtras,* by Swami Jyotirmayananda,** published by Yoga Research Foundation.

Swami Jyotir Mayananda is one of the last living disciples of Master Swami Shivananda of Rishikesh, India. He has been based in Florida for many decades. In 1970, it was Swamiji who bestowed the name of Rama upon me and initiated me into *yoga* and Vedanta studies. I studied his book *Raja Yoga*, which was really the study of the *sūtras*. His work has inspired me ever since. His book gives a sweeping overview of the *sūtras*, extrapolating the important aspects that anyone can apply to their lives. His knowledge is so vast that he can distill and simplify concepts into the language of this era. His work is truly brilliant in the ways he integrates our life's situations into the ancient teachings. The definition of a master is one who takes something difficult and makes it appear simple. Swamiji is truly a master in how he makes everything understandable using parables and people's experiences as examples in the teachings. It was Swamiji who created the charts of the chariot and four parts of mind, the varying stages of the *kleshas*, and the Wheel and Tree of Karma. I have adapted these charts to this book giving credit to him, not just for the charts but also for his teachings that will forever remain with me and continue to inspire me so that I may pass that inspiration onto others. Even though I have not seen him for many years, I will always think of him as my teacher who set my feet on the path of the *Yoga Sūtras*.

***The Yoga Sūtras of Patañjali,* by Swami Satchidananda,** published by Integral Yoga.

This is one of the most clear, concise, and accurate translations of *Patañjali's Yoga Sūtras*. Swamiji has a wonderful way of simplifying even the most complex areas of scripture by relating it to parables of the past and to our lives. This version is a great companion to the version of Swami Hariharinanda because Swamiji gives the meaning of each verb of Sanskrit and then gives the phonetic translation. Swami Hariharananda's version has only the Sanskrit Devanagari script and the English translation. Swamiji's book is necessary for one who wants to pronounce the *sūtras* phonetically according to the Sanskrit diacritical markings.

Swami Satchidananda however does not tackle the very esoteric translations of the third chapter so there is very little commentary, but he gives accurate translations and pronunciations. He was always a great storyteller. It is obvious in the way he threads stories throughout the *sūtras* that help us understand even the most complex concepts. Many years ago, he was visiting my home at Christmas time and I arranged for a gathering of *yoga* teachers to come and greet him. He sat in front of the huge Christmas tree with his long white hair and beard looking like a cross between Jesus Christ and Santa Clause. He gave an inspiring message and joked and laughed with us. One teacher then asked, "You seem so light hearted about *yoga*. Isn't it a serious subject?" He stroked his long white beard and said slowly, "Hum, light ... in light ... hum ... en-light-en-ment. Isn't that what *yoga* is about?"

His book is with me always and through it, I feel his beloved presence and his unforgettable and unending inspiration.

***Light on the Yoga Sūtras of Patañjali,* by B.K.S. Iyengar** (various publishers).

What gifts Mr. Iyengar has given to the world! He has given the gift of alignment that goes far beyond the physical body, and the gift of the *Yoga Sūtras*. This translation and commentaries are brilliant, because he integrates this ancient philosophy into the tenants of the *yoga* practices. In 1970, I sought out Mr. Iyengar in India because it was difficult to believe that the man pictured in the newly published book, *Light on Yoga* was the same man speaking about the philosophy in his book. I always believed that the practice of *asana* was inseparable from the philosophy, and for decades Mr. Iyengar has been paving the way for others to see how the *yoga* philosophy is woven in to the practices of *asana* and *pranayama*. In his book, he gives the Sanskrit and English translations, which integrate the vastness of the *sūtras* with the awareness of the physical body. It is extraordinary! It has been a long time since he was insistent that I have Swami Hariharananda's translation, and Mr. Iyengar's book does not seem to draw upon that interpretation. Instead, it was the springboard for his commentaries from his years of teaching that reflected his vast knowledge of the integration of the individuated microcosmic universe of our physical and subtle body with the universal macrocosm of the stars and planets of the cosmos.

***The Yoga Sūtras of Patañjali: A Study Guide for Book I & II,* by Baba Hari Dass.** Sri Rama Publishing.

I've known Babaji since the first time he came to this country. In the later years of the 1960s-70s, a handful of us would hang out with him in his room and simply ask questions. He had taken a vow of *mouna,* or silence, and would communicate through hand gestures and writing on a little blackboard he suspended like a necklace over his heart center. He was tireless as he wrote answers to our every question. I asked him so many questions about the *Yoga Sūtras*, and he answered not just the questions, but also the origins of the questions. Babaji was a true *yogin*. He answered in brief, succinct sentences that never went over the boundaries of his small blackboard. He was so eager to share his wisdom and insights with us that he infused us with the power of the "unspoken" word. He taught so much through his silence. Even though he silently taught the *sūtras* to his students, they were not put into a book form until decades later.

Babaji's version of the *sūtras* is also inspired by Swami Hariharananda Aranya. He used to quote from the Swamiji when giving classes on the *sūtras*. Babaji has left a wonderful legacy for future generations of *yogins* through his translation of scriptures and his presence of being. His version of *Patañjali's Yoga Sūtras* is divided into four chapters (books) that came out of dialogues with his devotees.

***The Heart of Yoga,* by T.K.V. Desikachar**, Inner Traditions.

Sri T.K.V Desikachar continued the legacy of his father, Sri T. Krishnamacharya, the great *yogi* and Sanskrit scholar. Desikachar was masterful in his ability to bring the *sūtras* into the understanding of everyday life. Again, he was impressive in the way he could take the most difficult concepts and make them understandable to mild as well as intense students of *yoga*. I remember sitting on the rooftop of his home in India with a gentle breeze blowing as he spoke of the *sūtras* and elicited questions from those of us who were there to inhale his knowledge.

I would not have had the courage to do this book on my understanding of the *Yoga Sūtras* if it were not for Desikachar. He was insistent that I leave the legacy of my many years in *yoga* and resulting experiences for future generations. The legacy he has left behind in the afterglow of his life on earth is invaluable to our *yoga* world. As a householder, he truly lived and integrated the *sūtras* into every phase of his life and teachings. What a gift he has given to us all in the legacy *he* has left for all future generations of *yogins*! His teachings continue through his family.

***The Yoga Sūtras of Patañjali,* by Swami Veda Bharati** (out of print)

This is truly a great treatise on the *Yoga Sūtras*. Swamiji was a disciple of Swami Rama of the Himalayan Institute both in the United States and India. Swami Veda, as we called him, was truly a great soul who is a living testament to the teachings of *yoga* and meditation. His book is as huge as his consciousness. In it, the pages are filled with the accurate translations and reflect the vastness of his wisdom and knowledge as a great master. He spent his final years in seclusion in India. Even though he withdrew from the world in meditation, he immensely benefited our world. Even though he is not well known in the popular world of *yoga* today, the legacy of his work through his students and his writing will shed light on the path of *yoga* well into this third millennium. What a great soul! I am so blessed to have known him, for through his presence he has blessed my life and given greater understanding of *yoga*.

***The Secret of the Yoga Sūtras,* by Pandit Rajmani Tigunait,** Himalayan Institute Press.

Wow! Panditiji, a disciple of Swami Rama, founder of the Himalayan Institute, was a Gurubai of Swami Veda Bharati. Panditiji is continuing the work of the Institute through his teachings and his writings. His book on the *Yoga Sūtras Chapter One* relates *yoga* to all aspects of life. It is written from his heart as well as experiences and I recommend it for giving students a feeling and deeper appreciation of the *sūtras*.

The following is a list of books that were written by friends of mine who are the first and second generation of American yogins to teach here in the United States. They come from a variety of lineages and have given a great gift to the world through their teachings and their presence. Their devotion to Yoga is obvious through their writings, which will remain as a legacy for generations to come.

***The Secret Power of Yoga,* by Nischala Joy Devi,** Three Rivers Press.

This is a woman's guide to the heart and spirit of the *Yoga Sūtras*. Her wonderful summary of the *sūtras* and how they apply to the ancient philosophy as well as issues that women, and men, contend with in our world of today. It is beautifully written from a woman's perspective but is universal in its content. Nischala has been in the *yoga* world since it first began its popular entrance into the United States. She travels the world giving workshops. Her book reflects a life steeped in *yoga* and a person who lives its philosophy.

***Yoga Sūtras of Patañjali,* by Mukunda Stiles,** Weiser Books.

Even though Mukunda is in *Mahasamādhi*, his work lives on. He wrote wonderful books, *Structural Yoga Therapy*, *Ayurveda and Yoga Therapy*, and commentaries on the *sūtras*. In his small book on the *Yoga Sūtras*, he kept his commentaries as short as the aphorisms of Patañjali. He distilled the *sūtras* down to their smallest common denominator. They are an accurate, and heartfelt legacy, and will be read and remembered in the *yoga* world by future generations. He was deeply dedicated to his studying, teaching and writing and that comes through the illuminations of his written words and his memory.

***The Yogi's Roadmap: Patañjali Yoga Sūtra as a Journey to Self Realization*, by Bhavani Silvia Maki,** Viveka Press.

Bhavani worked closely with her Ashtanga Yoga teacher Pattabhi Jois in India, for many years. She is a Bhakti *yogini* with a heart that embraces all beings. She is the daughter of a linguist and took immediately to Sanskrit after being introduced to the teachings of the *sūtras*. She was ignited with the fervor of the scriptures as if she was remembering that which she always knew. She beautifully weaves the *yoga* practice of *asana* into its philosophy and into one's life. All who have read her book are touched by her heartfelt devotion to *yoga* that leaps through the pages to ignite inspiration in the reader. As she says, "It is a 'roadmap,' not just to enlightenment but for the way we can live our lives."

***The Yoga Sūtra Workbook,* by Vyaas Houston,** founder of the American Sanskrit Institute.

I met Vyaas in San Francisco in the 1960s when he was studying with Dr. Ramamurti Mishra (Swami Brahmananda), a medical doctor and Sanskrit scholar who wrote a magnificent treatise on the psychology of yoga. The Indian doctor would say that the philosophy of the *Yoga Sūtras* is the deepest form of psychology in our world today. Dr. Mishra was also a scholar of Sanskrit. He taught Sanskrit for many hours daily to his devotees. Vyass lived in the *ashram* and received the transmission and love of this ancient language from his teacher Dr. Mishra. Vyaas has inspired thousands of people over the years with his teachings, and development of ever evolving teaching methodologies.

Vyaas has a new *Yoga Sūtras Workbook* and a *Sanskrit Atlas* edition. He shares insights and practices that emerged from his love and study of the Sanskrit language. His revised *Yoga Sūtras Workbooks* and *Panini Atlas* are born from his own deep personal study of Sanskrit as a practice of *yoga*. Vyass says, "The study of the language itself is the practice of yoga." His lifetime of experiential studies is vast where he intimates that, "internalized by meditation, the definitions of Patañjali become a living experience."

***The Yoga Sūtras: An Essential Guide to the Heart of Yoga Philosophy*, by Nicolai Bachman,** Sounds True, Inc.

Nicolai studied Sanskrit for many years with a longtime friend of mine, Vyaas Houston. The philosophy of the Yoga Sūtras is the deepest form of psychology in our world today. Nicolai carries on the transmission of the lineage of Dr. Mishra and Vyass in his own path and has given the world a beautiful work of the *sūtras*. He does not go *sutra*-by-*sūtra*, but compiles them into interrelated groupings that help the reader to understand how varying *sūtras* interrelate and can be woven together. Nicolai's book is magnificently packaged. There is the spiral bound *sūtra* book, CDs and a DVD to listen to while traveling along with flash cards. I think this is a must for every *yoga* library. It is not only beautiful to look at, it is filled with the knowledge of the ages.

***The Science of Yoga*, by I.K. Taimni** (various publishers)

I did not know him personally, but this was one of the first books I studied on the *Yoga Sūtras* in the 1960s. It is clear in its description and is exoteric in its explanations, so it can be immediately applied to everyday life. There is not too much that one can find objectionable or "too far out." He has a wonderful way of simplifying and putting complex concepts into a form that most anyone can understand. It is a good book that has stood the test of time and continues to be a reliable study guide for students taking the early steps into the infinite ocean of the *Yoga Sūtras*.

The Yoga Sūtra books we choose to guide us through the commentaries are important for our understanding. The following is a list of additional books on the Yoga Sūtras that are currently available.

Baba, Bangali. *Yogasūtra of Patañjali: With the Commentary of Vyasa*. 1976. Motilal Banarsidass Publishers Pvt. Ltd. Delhi, India.

Bouanchaud, Bernard. *The Essence of Yoga.* 1997. Rudra Press. Portland, OR.

Bryant, Edwin F. *The Yoga Sūtras of Patañjali.* 2009. North Point Press. New York, NY.

Christensen, Alice. *Yoga of the Heart.* 1998. Daybreak Books. New York, NY.

Desikachar, T.K.V. *Patañjali's Sūtras: An Introduction.* 1987. Affiliated East-West Press Pvt. Ltd. New Delhi, India.

Desikachar, T.K.V. *Reflections on Yoga Sūtra-s of Patañjali.* revised 2003. Krishnamacharya Yoga Mandiram. Chennai, India.

Feuerstein, Georg. *The Yoga Sūtras of Patañjali.* 1989. Inner Traditions International. Rochester, VT.

Govindan, Marshall. *Kriya Yoga Sūtras of Patañjali and the Siddhas.* 2000. Kriya Yoga Publications. Quebec, Canada.

Hartranft, Chip. *The Yoga-Sūtra of Patañjali.* 2003. Shambhala Publications. Boston, MA.

Krishnamacharya, Sri. T. *Pantajalyaogadarsanam.* 1999. Krishnamacharya Yoga Mandiram. Chennai, India.

MSI. *Enlightenment! The Yoga Sutras.* 1996. Society for Ascension. Waynesville, FL.

McClure, Vimala. *The Ethics of Love,* 1992. Nucleus Publications. Willow Springs, MO.

Nelson, Sonia. *Patañjali's Yoga Sūtras, A Chanting Tutorial.* 2002. ViaMedia Productions. Santa Fe, NM.

Prabhavananda, Swami, and Isherwood, Christopher. *How to Know God.* 1981. Vedanta Press. Hollywood, California.

Prasada, Rama, *Patañjali's Yoga Sūtras*. 1912. Munshiram Manoharlal Publishers Pvt. Ltd. New Delhi, India.

Saraswati, Swami Satyananda. *Four Chapters on Freedom.* 1997. Yoga Publications Trust. Munger, Bihar, India.

Schubert, Jeffery. *Yoga Sūtra's of Patañjali.* 2002. Self published. Evergreen, CO.

Shearer, Alistair. *The Yoga Sūtras of Patañjali.* 1982. Bell Tower. New York, NY.

Tigunait, Pandit Rajmani. *The Practice of the Yoga Sūtra: Sadhana Pada.* 2017. Himalayan Institute, Honesdale, PA.

Tigunait, Pandit Rajmani. *The Secret of the Yoga Sūtras.* 2015. Himalayan Institute Press. Honesdale, PA.

Venkatesananda, Swami. *The Yoga Sūtras of Patañjali.* 2008. Motilal. Banarsidass, Dehli, India.

Zambita, Salvatore. *The Unadorned Thread of Yoga*, 1992. The Yoga-Sūtras Institute Press. Poulsbo, WA.

Guide to Pronunciations

	Devanagari/ Transliteration	Pronunciation	Meaning
Vowels			
Guttural	अ *a*	as in **A**merica	
	आ *ā*	as in f**a**ther	
Palatal	इ *i*	as in h**i**ll	
	ई *ī*	as in sl**ee**p	
Dental	उ *u*	as in p**u**t	
	ऊ *ū*	as in r**u**de	
Guttural	ए *e*	as in pr**e**y	
	ऐ *ai*	as in as in **ai**sle	
Dental	ओ *o*	as in g**o**	
	औ *au*	as in **ou**t	
Cerebral	ऋ *ṛ*	as in ma**rin**	
	ॠ *ṝ*	as in ma**rine**	
Dental	ऌ *ḷr*	as in a**lr**ight	
	ॡ *ḹr*	as in **all-r**eaching	
Anusvara	अं *aṅ/añ/aṇ/an/aṃ*	as in pl**um, sun,** ru**ng**, etc.	
Visarga	अः *aḥ*	as in **haha**	
Consonants			
Guttural	क *ka*	as in **cu**t	Interrogation, diminution, action
	ख *kha*	as in **kh**an	The sky, heavens, celestial worlds
	ग *ga*	as in **gu**ttural	To go, commence, start, etc.
	घ *gha*	as in **gh**ost	To smell, denseness, high frequency odors
	ङ *ṅa*	as in go**ng**	A part, section, piece
Palatal	च *ca*	as in **ch**ipper	Conjunction, reinforcement, reduplication
	छ *cha*	as in mu**ch-h**am	Shadow, darkness, shelter

	ज *ja*	as in **j**ug	Birth, Creation, Wisdom, re-birth
	झ *jha*	as in hed**ge-h**og	Warring enemies of Spirit
	ञ *ña*	as in o**n-y**acht	Knowledge, understanding
Cerebral	ट *ṭa*	as in bor**scht**	Spiritual pride
	ठ *ṭha*	as in an**t-h**ill	Flourish, explosive
	ड *ḍa*	as in yar**d**	Tumult, chaos, commotion
	ढ *ḍha*	as in re**d-h**ill	Vagueness, obscure, to disappear
	ण *ṇa*	as in ea**rn**est	Cosmic vibratory inflow of undifferentiated ideation
Dental	त *ta*	as in **t**ouch	*Suchness, activation*
	थ *tha*	as in ea**t-h**ummus	Dwelling, a place, relating, The Moon
	द *da*	as in **d**ental	Generosity, Creation, Giving
	ध *dha*	as in en**d-h**unger	The realm of the Dharma, position
	न *na*	as in **n**othing	Negation, name, cognition
Labial	प *pa*	as in **p**apa	Paternal, Male aspect, ultimate
	फ pha	as in u**p-h**ill	Flower, blossom, grow, foam
	ब *ba*	as in **b**abaganoush	To bind, to relate
	भ *bha*	as in a**bh**or	Creation, Creator, Existence, transcension
	म *ma*	as in **m**other	Mother, Female aspect, to measure, my/mine
Semi-vowels (consonants derived from Vowels)			
Palatal	य *ya*	as in **y**ard	To activate, commence, a vehicle, Bījam
Cerebral	र *ra*	as in **R**ama	Passion, growth, The Sun, Bījam
Labial	ल *la*	as in **l**ove	To mark, dissolve, ascend, Bījam
Dental	व va	as in **v**anilla	To speak, to relate, Bījam
Sibilants			
Palatal	श *śa*	as in **sh**ut	Peace, Beatitude, Regeneration
Cerebral	ष *ṣa*	as in **sch**napps	The senses, sense organs, Fire
Dental	स *sa*	as in **s**erpent	Truth, Hissing, Goodness, Happiness
Aspirant	ह *ha*	as in **h**ot	The Sun, growth, Causation, prāṇa

www.ingramcontent.com/pod-product-compliance
Lightning Source LLC
Chambersburg PA
CBHW081356290426
44110CB00018B/2400